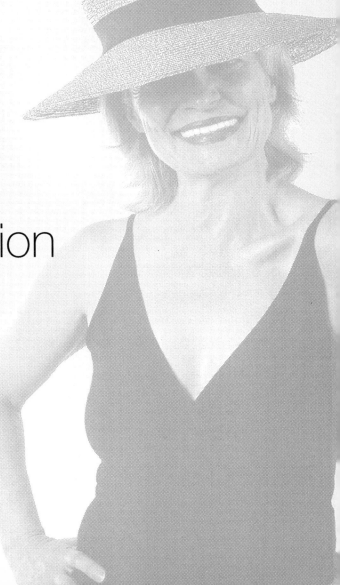

Step 1

Health
information

Many women approaching or experiencing menopause are confused and frustrated with the information available to them on how best to manage this stage of their life. With or without hormone replacement therapy (HRT) a simple lifestyle plan is needed to give women the autonomy to take control of their menopause. Research reveals that certain lifestyle behaviours have positive effects on menopausal symptoms, but an ad hoc approach is still being used by many women. Our lifestyle plan consists of six steps that women can take to minimise menopausal symptoms and maximise the quality of their life into the future. This new *Menopause Made Simple Program* will benefit all menopausal women, regardless of whether they are using HRT.

What can I expect at menopause? How will my body change? These are normal questions that every woman wants answered as she approaches or experiences menopause. This section describes the changes that happen in your body at this time of life and explores what you can, and cannot, expect at menopause. We discuss the common symptoms that women might experience during menopause in Western culture and in other cultures.

We explore how meaningful your attitude and expectations of menopause are to your own journey and discuss the importance of seeking out accurate health information about menopause for yourself.

The
Menopause
Made Simple
Program

Dr Debra Anderson PhD is a senior lecturer in women's health and nursing at the Queensland University of Technology. She has held executive positions including Chair of Women's Health Queensland Wide, and is a member of the Australasian, Asia–Pacific and International Menopause societies. She conducted her doctorate in the area of menopause and is currently chief investigator on the Queensland Women's Midlife Study and the Australian and Japanese Cross Cultural Menopause Study.

Vicky Graham BHMS B Bus is an outstanding exercise physiologist and teacher who specialises in menopausal women. She has been involved in the health and fitness industry for over 15 years, teaching a wide range of people from children to adolescents through to adults. Vicky's ability to provide practical advice and ideas to help achieve a healthier lifestyle has been appreciated by the many women that she has worked with to date.

The Menopause Made Simple Program

Maximise your lifestyle by
minimising your symptoms

**Dr Debra Anderson
and Vicky Graham**

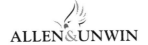

ALLEN&UNWIN

First published in 2002

Allen & Unwin
83 Alexander Street
Crows Nest NSW 2065
Australia
Phone: (61 2) 8425 0100
Fax: (61 2) 9906 2218
Email: info@allenandunwin.com
Web: www.allenandunwin.com

National Library of Australia
Cataloguing-in-Publication entry:

Anderson, Debra, 1961– .
  The menopause made simple program: maximise your lifestyle
  by minimising your symptoms.

  Bibliography.
  Includes index.
  ISBN 1 86508 767 X.

  1. Menopause—Popular works. 2. Women—Health and
  hygiene. 3. Menopause—Treatment—Popular works.
  4. Menopause—Nutritional aspects—Popular works. 5. Diet.
  I. Graham, Vicky, 1966– . II. Title.

612.665

Text design by Simon Paterson
Internal photographs by Dave Bredeson
Set in 11/14 pt Caslon by Bookhouse, Sydney
Printed in Australia by McPherson's Printing Group

10 9 8 7 6 5 4 3 2 1

Contents

Step 1: Health information   **1**
1   Knowledge   3
2   Expectations   8
3   Bodily changes   12
4   Menopausal symptoms   18
5   General health   25

Step 2: Eating for menopause   **37**
6   A healthy eating plan   39
7   Dietary considerations for menopause   47
8   Weight control   58

Step 3: Exercising for menopause   **71**
9   The benefits of exercise   73
10   Choosing your exercise   84
11   Pelvic floor exercises   103
12   How to get started   108

Step 4: Hormone replacement therapy   **121**
13   HRT: to use or not to use?   123
14   Short-term use vs long-term use   129
15   HRT: risks and benefits   135

Step 5: Alternatives to HRT   **147**
16   Complementary therapies   149
17   Supplements   154

Step 6: Putting it into practice   **165**
18   The Menopause Made Simple Program   167
19   The Menopause Made Simple Program Journal   171

Appendix: Long-term studies into HRT use   215
Endnotes   217
Further reading   219
Bibliography   220
Index   225

Don't wait for a light to appear at the end of the tunnel.
Stride down there... and light the bloody thing yourself.

Sara Henderson

Chapter 1

Knowledge

If you are reading this book you are probably one of the 476 million women worldwide currently going through menopause or one of the many others approaching this time of life. Why has menopause suddenly become so topical? Hardly a week goes by without some aspect of menopause, hormone replacement therapy or alternatives to HRT being mentioned in the media. The information is so conflicting that it's difficult to make the right decisions. One article tells you that HRT is good for the heart; another warns that it will give you breast cancer. A TV program suggests that menopause is all in your head; another claims that your natural ageing process is a medical condition that needs to be treated. Confusion reigns.

As a doctoral researcher for close to four years, I have immersed myself in menopause and HRT and its alternatives, reviewing the literature, interviewing women and exploring their views and experiences throughout menopause. I have led studies that compared Australian and Asian women and am currently working closely with researchers from Japan and Taiwan to try to unlock the mysteries surrounding menopause across the globe.

Vicky Graham has had extensive professional practice with women who are going through menopause or searching for information about it. As an exercise physiologist specialising in menopausal women, Vicky has developed personal lifestyle programs for women to help them achieve their goals during and after menopause. *The Menopause Made Simple Program* is the result of our working together to design a program based both on research and on the life experiences of women.

It is this information that we would like to share with you. We offer you the most recently researched information on menopause and suggest a way to package all this information into a lifestyle program, to ensure that your menopause is what you want it to be. Along the way we share some of the experiences that women from both Western and non-Western countries have described to us in our professional practice and studies that we hope will relate to your own experiences or expectations of menopause. Women have told us that this is what they want...

> *...to call up the right information and information that women can understand. As we're all at different levels of education, you want something that's pure and simple, a couple of books that you can read. Nothing too thick; you just need information which is simple and not extended and not too long.*

That is our aim—to work with you and provide you with clear, well researched facts about menopause. The information available is extensive and confusing; we hope to simplify it so that you can use it to take control of your own journey through menopause.

Let's define menopause.

Menopause is that time of life when menstruation (or periods) stops and usually occurs between the ages of 45 and 54 years. It is a time when the hormones change and the level of oestrogen starts to decline slowly.

Most women feel relieved when menopause comes, and report very few changes in their feelings and state of mind or body. However, about 20 per cent of women have a hard time during menopause and experience quite overwhelming changes. We don't know why this is so, but I liken it to the days of premenstrual tension (PMT): in a group of six girls, four would hardly notice that their periods were coming, but two would know for about a week before, experiencing all sorts of bodily changes, from bloated breasts to depression and teariness. A small number found that PMT seriously disrupted their life. And so it appears with menopause: some women sail through it, saying, 'I didn't even notice it', and some women get a few changes which they feel confident in handling themselves. A few women, however, get severe changes and symptoms and benefit from the support of health professionals.

There don't seem to be any hard and fast rules, although you may gain a little insight from your mother or sisters—in some families there seems to be a tendency to breeze through menopause or to be badly affected by it.

Menopause: changing perceptions

The menopausal woman is not normal; she suffers from a deficiency disease with serious sequelae and needs treatment. (Wilson, Brevetti and Wilson, 1963)

A large percentage of women ... acquire a vapid cowlike feeling called a 'negative state'. It is a strange endogenous misery ... the world appears as though through a grey veil, and they live as docile, harmless creatures missing most of life's values. (Wilson and Wilson, 1963)

That quotation is actually taken from a medical textbook. It would be hard to imagine someone writing that today but negative expectations surrounding menopause have been recorded throughout history. This extreme view of the menopausal woman was eventually discarded, although some authors and media and health professionals still reflect some aspects of it.

More recent studies have helped to expel the myths surrounding menopause, although the experience of women during this phase of life remains a mystery for many people. Menopause needs to be understood in the context of today. By portraying menopausal women in this negative light—and in the process convincing them they have a serious problem that must be treated—society is able to ensure that menopause becomes and remains big business. You need to keep this in mind as you explore the enormous amount of conflicting material and advice that surrounds this issue.

There are several reasons why menopause is treated in the way it is today. The focus on the health of middle-aged women in the society of the last century would have been insignificant because most women died before 40 years of age. Today, however, women live to an average age of 79 years and health care for older women is considered important. The focus on health care for menopausal women can be seen as a phenomenon of the 1900s.

According to the World Health Organization, the average age of menopause is 50 years. It can be calculated that one in every two to three women can expect to live for more than 30 years after menopause. That's a lot of women experiencing menopause. It is important that we get right the information on health care for women over the age of 45 years.

Baby boomers and menopause

The baby boomers have a lot to answer for. The generation of women following them will, in time, I feel, be grateful for the advances that they demanded and received for women in the area of health care. To begin with, the baby boomers pushed for women to have the choice to work outside the home, and won. Second, they demanded that women have choices in reproductive health, and won. This generation of women fought long and hard to ensure that women could choose the way they gave birth. No longer was childbirth to be seen as a medical condition that needed to be treated; rather, it was a partnership of mother, father and health professionals working together to ensure that, where possible, women could have their choice of birth. Another tick for the baby boomers is that they reorientated health care by promoting and demanding health care that was more woman-centred.

And how does this relate to menopause? I believe that the baby boomers are doing it again. In the twentieth century, menopause was treated and portrayed as a medical condition in need of treatment. Various drugs and therapies were developed and prescribed for women going through this phase of life. Menopause has been treated as an oestrogen deficiency disease—the stereotypical view of menopausal women has been a woman with a deficit disease who is described as experiencing a large range of symptoms and being a great user of the medical system.

Here are two women's experiences of their consultations for menopause in the 1990s.

The doctors don't tell you anything. They don't say, go to your library and read this book. And they don't give you any alternatives—it seems like they've catalogued everybody.

It's like being on a merry-go-round of referral from one doctor to another doctor and, unless you know the questions to ask, you don't get an answer.

However, the baby boomers are changing forever the way that menopause is treated and viewed. The changes are slow, but there is a strong ground swell of women in their forties and fifties who refuse to be told that the time of life called menopause is something to be feared. As consumers of the health care system, they are demanding, informed choices in the way they experience this time of life. Women from this generation have access to an enormous amount of information that was previously unavailable, and they also have the confidence to look for it and use it. In the new millennium a baby boomer's consultation on menopause may go something like this:

'Doctor, I've researched information on hormone replacement therapy and alternatives to HRT and I was wondering if we can work out together the best program for me, considering my family background in heart disease, breast cancer and osteoporosis.'

Watch out as the baby boomers handle menopause their way and pave the way for a new era in menopausal health care for future generations of women!

Chapter 2

Expectations

Women should be taught about menopause before they reach menopause, so that they're aware of what's going to happen. (Janet)

When it comes to menopause there is evidence to suggest that what you expect is what you get. Research supports the notion of a self-fulfilling prophecy and suggests that how a woman experiences menopause may be related more to what the woman is like than to the condition itself.

Most women say they are relieved, or they don't really feel strongly about menopause and this finding seems to be true across both time and cultures. Most women simply feel relief when their periods stop rather than an overwhelming loss.

Menopause has different meanings for women from different countries. In India and Southern Asia, for example, it is viewed as a positive event, an end to taboos and social restrictions. It is also positive in Greek and Japanese cultures—in fact, it is given little thought. The most positive attitude is held by Arab countries, where menopause is closely related to the freedom of having no more children. Unfortunately, the view that we are most familiar with is that of Western countries, which see menopause as a deficiency disease.

Many well constructed studies have been conducted with women from these countries and the research findings clearly show that *the way women experience menopause differs from country to country and particularly between Western and non-Westernised countries.*

What is happening here?

Is it *diet*? Western and non-Western women have very different approaches to diet: Western women tend to consume high levels of fat and only small amounts of grain while Asian women, for example, consume large amounts of grains, fresh vegetables and soy products. These foods contain high levels of a plant-based oestrogen called phytoestrogen and some scientists believe this may be one of the reasons for the differences seen across cultures. We examine phytoestrogens in detail in Step 2, *Eating for menopause*, to enable you to decide whether you want to increase them in your diet.

Is it *society's attitudes to women*? In non-Western countries, women are viewed with esteem as they get older, while women in Western countries tend to experience ageism, finding that older women are not valued as highly as they should be.

Is it *genetics*? Are women from non-Western countries programmed differently to experience menopause in different ways?

Or is it *lifestyle*? Women in Western countries often have very different lifestyle patterns to non-Western women, with different approaches to self-help health measures, exercise, social supports, spirituality and working patterns. Taiwanese women described their approach to menopause in this way:

> *Have exercise, leisure activity, and sleep well. Besides maintaining the balance of your mood as well as your diet, take your menopause lightly but face those physical changes bravely, and live as you used to live.*

> *Maintain regular exercise, build up a positive philosophy of life and learn the techniques to relax yourself.* [1]

We don't know the answer yet, but research continues to be undertaken in this important area. What we do know is that there is a lot to learn from each other across the cultures, when women share their stories and what works for them in different parts of the world. We are continuing our studies comparing women from Western and non-Western

Food for thought

Much of the early research on menopause was conducted in what are called 'clinical trials'. This type of research uses samples of women who come into clinics, and excludes women in the general population. Women who attend clinics are usually there for a particular problem. Studies like these exclude the 'well' menopausal woman who has not visited a clinic because she doesn't feel a need. This restricted selection has been a tremendous problem in the research conducted on menopausal women. To get around this problem the World Health Organization has recommended that, where possible, further menopause studies should be conducted on the general population of women so that all women in the community are represented, not just those attending clinics. When you are looking at reported research on menopause, a key question that you should ask yourself is: On what type of women was this study conducted? Because of the way that clinical trials are conducted, it is largely unknown whether menopausal complaints in the general population are actually due to menopause, or to the natural ageing process, or other social or psychological factors in a woman's life.

countries to ensure that precious information on women's health from all parts of the world can be shared and made available to all.

Outside influences on the menopausal experience

Many things, other than your oestrogen levels (hormones), can affect the way that you experience menopause. All these are important and legitimate, and it does appear that your experience of menopause is associated with the many roles that you may play in life as a woman.

Researchers have found many elements that may impact on your menopause and the symptoms you feel, including your personality, lifestyle, stress levels, social support, education level, and whether you are working full-time, part-time or at home.[2]

The findings suggest that the most helpful strategies for menopausal women are those that improve your general health, increase positive lifestyle behaviours and foster positive attitudes towards menopause and ageing. These strategies have been incorporated into *The Menopause Made Simple Program* with guidelines on diet, exercise, health and other options to enhance the experience of menopause and beyond.

Chapter 3

Bodily changes

I think if people treated it as normal, not abnormal, then we'd be able to cope with it better. (Susan)

Menopause brings changes to the body that are unwelcome to some women. But it's important to remember that, although periods cease for all women at the onset of menopause, the various 'symptoms' of menopause occur in only a minority of women.

Dennerstein and colleagues argue that there are several factors which make women more or less likely to experience menopausal symptoms. They found that women who are less likely to have menopausal symptoms:

- have a higher level of education;
- rate their self-health highly;
- have no chronic health conditions;
- experience low personal stress;
- have no previous premenstrual compaints;
- do not smoke;
- exercise at least once a week;
- have a positive attitude towards menopause and ageing.

Those who are more likely to experience menopausal symptoms:

- have a lower level of education;
- rate their self-health low;
- have one or more chronic health conditions;
- suffer high personal stress;
- have previous premenstrual compaints;
- smoke;
- do not exercise;
- have a negative attitude towards menopause and ageing.[2]

Education

So to begin with, what we want to do is eliminate as many of these variables as possible before we look at the changes that may take place in our bodies. Let's start with education. You may feel you cannot change your level of education, but just by reading this book you are increasing your *knowledge* about menopause. Women with a better education are more likely to seek out information about their health, and that is why seeking out health information about menopause is the first step in *The Menopause Made Simple Program*. Knowledge will empower you to take control of your menopause.

Self-rated health

How healthy do you think you are? This assessment is called your self-rated health and often goes hand in hand with self-esteem. When you perceive yourself as healthy, you tend to act in that way. There is a theory that states: 'the more positive health behaviours you engage in, the more you are likely to engage in, and so it goes on.' Juliet's story demonstrates this theory.

It does appear that just by starting one positive health behaviour (e.g. exercise) you are very likely to start another and another, and in the process increase your self-rated health.

That is why we have included a comprehensive approach for you to use during menopause. We know that if you take the first step, *Health*

Juliet is 53 years old and a heavy smoker. She does not exercise and has a typical Western diet, high in saturated fat. Juliet feels depressed and describes herself as having little energy.

Juliet began a walking program. Starting very slowly, she walked to the end of the street and back and then found herself looking forward to walking every day until she was driving herself to a shady park, where she found a 5 km circuit which she walked comfortably. Juliet's energy levels increased and she described herself as not feeling depressed. Juliet surprised herself at what she could achieve and she thought, if I can do this I can stop smoking. Juliet chose New Year's Day to quit smoking and has (with the aid of her pharmacist) continued this positive health behaviour. Juliet's self-rated health has increased again and she began to feel like eating healthy, nutritious foods instead of her usual high-fat diet. She also started to apply sunscreen while walking and her self-rated health went up even higher.

information (which you already have, by purchasing this book), you are very likely to take the next five steps as well.

Chronic health conditions and previous premenstrual complaints

This is an area that is largely beyond your control. The important thing is to ensure that you have a good health professional to advise you on the best treatment possible. Remember, too, that seeking out health information can help you feel more in control of your disorder so that, instead of the condition taking over your life, you live with it to the best of your ability.

There are many good websites available, covering all sorts of conditions. Just type in the condition under 'Search' and you will be surprised what you come up with. Some sites are better than others, so be discerning about which website you take your information from.

Have a look at who is sponsoring the website and who is writing it. An excellent website for women to obtain credible, well-researched information is the Harvard Women's Health Watch at www.health.harvard.edu /newsletters/whtext.html.

Stress

Stress seems to be linked to many health complaints, but we can take control of our stress. It seems that if you normally have lower rates of interpersonal stress, you are less likely to suffer from menopausal symptoms, and from poor health in general.

We all suffer from external stresses in our lives—spouses get angry, teenage children don't live their lives as we would like, or work colleagues don't support you. The trick is what we do with that stress, how we cope with it. It is called interpersonal stress and it is this stress that we allow to build up in our bodies.

It is vitally important that you learn how to deal with stress and process it in a meaningful way so that it does not accumulate and damage your body. This may be in the form of meditation, letting it all out (a big yell at the trees when no one else is around), exercising or learning to choose your reaction (i.e. consciously deciding that you will not get stressed over the matter). Whatever your strategy, decreasing and combating interpersonal stress in your life will be one of the most important things that you can do for your health now and into the future.

Why not consider using some of these stress management strategies?

- yoga
- relaxation and or meditation
- carving out time for yourself
- tai chi
- counselling and support.

Smoking

Many studies in different countries show that smoking increases the menopausal symptoms that women experience. Women who smoke are more likely to have an earlier menopause, around two years earlier than non-smokers. Women who smoke also describe their symptoms as more severe. We don't know the reason, but it does seem that smoking affects the physiology of the body and the hormones in the body.

Women who smoke also have increased wrinkling of the skin, particularly around the mouth and eyes, poorer physical health and lower self-rated health. There really are no positives that I can give you on smoking and menopause—if you plan to do anything for yourself in a positive way, try to cut out smoking. You will achieve more health benefits from this one positive behaviour than from anything else you can do for yourself. Seek the help of a health professional, and maybe speak to your pharmacist, to see if you can 'kick the habit'.

Exercise

While smoking is just about the *worst* thing you can do for your health as a woman, exercise is just about the *best* thing. Exercise will increase your self-rated health, may help to decrease your menopausal symptoms, and will improve your total health now and into the future. Research has found that exercise is the number one health behaviour required for decreasing menopausal symptoms and increasing the positive way that women feel about their health.[2]

For this reason we devote a whole section to *Exercising for menopause* (see Step 3). We have put together specific and important information and exercises for menopausal women, so that you can incorporate them into your everyday life. As women have told us:

> *I want specific information on exercise for women experiencing menopause. (Sandra)*

> *Exercise sessions for mature-aged women as well as relaxation exercises. (Pam)*

Attitude towards menopause and ageing

The more positive you feel about the menopause the less likely you are to experience menopausal symptoms. For example, although a positive attitude won't automatically get rid of hot flushes, it will probably make dealing with them easier.

Those of us who live in the Western world find that there is a heavy emphasis on youthful appearance and a slim figure. However, many women today refuse to accept the negative stereotypical image of the older woman that has been portrayed in the past. Menopause is not a time when you are sick or suffering, have a deficiency disease or need to be nurtured. Menopause today can be a time of empowerment, strength, vibrancy and fulfilment!

You can reverse many of the changes that we thought were inevitable. You can preserve bone density, improve the health of your heart and arteries and increase muscle strength and tone. You can take control of your menopause...and enjoy the journey!

Chapter 4

Menopausal symptoms

Symptoms involving all parts of the body have been attributed to menopause. It is difficult to determine which symptoms are due to menopause and which are due to the natural process of ageing.

The World Health Organization also found it perplexing, so much so that in 1996 they appointed a group of expert researchers from around the world to review all the available research and come up with the 'true' symptoms of menopause. They found that the following symptoms appear to be related to ageing, rather than to menopause itself, or can be associated with stress in mid-life. These symptoms are common to men as well as women.

- urinary problems
- depression
- nervous tension
- palpitations
- headaches
- insomnia
- lack of energy
- fluid retention
- backache
- difficulty in concentrating
- dizzy spells.

The WHO group named two 'true' symptoms of menopause—which included hot flushes and night sweats—as they were the symptoms most consistently associated with menopause.

Other symptoms that can be clearly linked to menopause include changes in the genital region and irregular periods in the 12 months leading up to their cessation.

The WHO group felt that the remaining symptoms were not necessarily specific to menopause and may in fact be psychological or related to a person's social or cultural group. These are symptoms like depression, nervous tension, palpitations, headaches, insomnia, lack of energy, fluid retention, backache, difficulty in concentration and dizzy spells. Now this does not mean that these symptoms are not real or important, but it does mean that they need to be treated differently, not all lumped together under the banner of menopause.

This WHO information is very useful for both health professionals and women themselves, so that the most appropriate treatment and strategies can be suggested for use during menopause.

Hot flushes and night sweats

Hot flushes and night sweats are 'thermoregulatory disturbances' that may occur during menopause. Think of your body as having a thermostat that keeps the body at a certain temperature. For some reason, during menopause, this thermostat sometimes gets out of control for a short period and the result is a hot flush or night sweat. Night sweats are just hot flushes that occur during the night, usually while you are asleep. Insomnia (not being able to sleep) is often linked to menopause as well, but it usually occurs as a result of night sweats that may happen while you are asleep. They may continually wake you up, so that you feel deprived of sleep.

Hot flushes usually last for up to three minutes. Women describe them as a sudden feeling of heat, usually occurring in the face, neck and chest region. Often there is patchy flushing of the skin in this area. You perspire a lot and you may get an uncomfortable feeling that your heart is beating fast (called a palpitation). Women report feeling quite uncomfortable during this process, and say that hot flushes occur more often when they are feeling tense or nervous.

Your likelihood of getting hot flushes and night sweats depends on a number of factors, as simple as which country you come from and whether you smoke. The World Health Organization found that these two symptoms are seen more consistently in women from European and North American origins (see graph below). Reasons for the differences shown in the graph are not yet known, but the WHO suggests that a high dietary intake of phytoestrogens in Japanese women, compared with Caucasian women, could be a possible explanation of their lower frequency of several symptoms.

The WHO report stated that phytoestrogens found in the urine were 110 times higher in Japanese women compared with Finnish women, and that the addition of phytoestrogens to a Western diet can produce positive changes of thickening in the lining of the vaginal walls.

Help for hot flushes

Oestrogens and/or progestogens (various forms of hormone replacement therapy) have been found to reduce the number and intensity of hot flushes. They seem to be equally effective in any of the forms available—tablets, patches or implants.

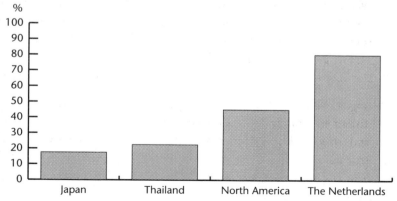

Percentage of women who experience hot flushes, selected countries

Source: WHO, 1996

20

Exercise—studies have shown that women who exercise during and after menopause have about half the number of severe hot flushes of women who don't.[4]

Paced respiration has also been shown to decrease the frequency of hot flushes.[5] Paced respiration is slow deep breathing. It goes like this... breathe in for five seconds, then slowly breathe out for five seconds. Now try to make the breath last a little longer. Breathe in for seven seconds and then slowly breathe out for seven seconds. The most effective time to start paced respiration is as soon as you feel the flush beginning—some women describe a tingling sensation in their fingers and toes at the beginning of a hot flush. Then do deep slow breathing for the duration of the hot flush. Many women say that paced respiration decreases the intensity of the flush and sometimes stops it in its tracks. You can do it anywhere—just quietly begin to take slow deep breaths and focus on your breathing.

This technique is recommended for women who experience hot flushes during menopause but do not wish or are unable to take HRT.

Changes in the vagina

After menopause the lining of the vagina becomes thinner, although this does not necessarily happen to all women. Even in old age, only about 20 per cent of women were found to have this change.[6]

The thinning of the vaginal wall can give you the feeling of a 'dry' vagina which can then become tender and sore, leading to difficulty in passing urine and uncomfortable intercourse. About 20 per cent of Australian women report this symptom, while only 4.5 per cent of women from Thailand mentioned this symptom.[7]

The following have been shown to help women with this change.

- *Oestrogen administration* (available in HRT)—effective in increasing the thickness and secretions of the vagina.
- *Vaginal lubricants*—offer reasonably effective non-hormonal treatment.
- *Continuing sexual activity*—may protect women against vaginal changes in menopause.

> ***Food for thought***
>
> Decreased sexual interest has been blamed on menopause, but recent studies have found that the decrease in interest was related more to the way the woman felt about her sexual partner and less to do with her menopause.
>
> *Source:* Dennerstein et al., 1993

- *Phytoestrogens*—research suggests that increasing these in your diet is effective in improving mild to moderate hot flushes.

Urinary problems

As women get older, problems with the waterworks become more widespread, occurring in 25–50 per cent of women. It is still unclear where we put the blame—on menopause, on the way our pregnancies and births were experienced or on the ageing process. Probably a combination of the three is likely.

Urinary problems that may occur include:

- a feeling of urgency to pass urine;
- pain when passing urine;
- having to get up to go to the toilet a lot at night;
- 'wetting your pants' when you sneeze, laugh or cough.

You can find help with urinary problems by consulting with a qualified health professional. Visit your general practitioner first, who will ensure that there is no urinary tract infection, and ask for a referral to a specialist nurse practitioner or specialist physiotherapist in the field. They will assess your situation and help you work towards full bladder control.

If you have urinary problems now in menopause, I strongly encourage you to get them sorted out, because they won't just go away and may get worse as you get older if you leave them untreated.

The good news is that in all cases you can achieve a big improvement. You do not need to live with any of these urinary problems.

Pelvic floor exercises

These exercises are covered in detail in Step 3, *Exercising for menopause*. They are important preventive exercises that you can do to keep the pelvic floor area strong and working for you.

Irregular bleeding during perimenopause

It is completely normal to experience changing menstrual patterns and irregular bleeding in the time coming up to menopause (perimenopause). Only about one in ten women stop bleeding abruptly. Most women have months and sometimes years of irregular cycles and bleeding at this time. This is quite normal—it is just your body adjusting to the changes occurring within it. The best treatment is not to worry about it and have faith that your body knows what it is doing.

Other complaints

As mentioned before, many symptoms are claimed to be part of menopause. I heard only yesterday an advertisement on the radio advertising a women's medical centre with the question: 'Is your menopause a misery?' This advertisement immediately suggests to women and the general public that menopausal women are meant to get depressed. Well, this just isn't true!

Let's get one thing clear—depression is not caused by menopause! Depression does not become more frequent at menopause than at other times. Depression is a serious condition that requires appropriate treatment and counselling from qualified health professionals.

Depression, nervous tension, palpitations, headaches, insomnia, lack of energy, fluid retention, backache, difficulty in concentrating and dizzy spells are not considered to be highly related to menopause. A study conducted in Holland, for example, found that none of these symptoms was more common among women than among men in the menopausal age range of 45–54 years.[8]

Most of the studies on hormone replacement therapy have found that HRT *does not* significantly help any of these problems. Treatment for these complaints needs to be conducted as it would be for anyone else. Consult with your general practitioner who will look for the real causes of the complaint and advise appropriate treatment.

Chapter 5

General health

The major cause of death in women over 65 years is not cancer but heart disease. Women are at greater risk of developing heart disease than breast cancer and dying from it in older age, yet women's greatest fear is of developing cancer, with breast cancer the most feared of all.

In this chapter we discuss some of the normal changes to your general health that may happen from menopause on. We focus on three aspects in particular—changes to the heart, changes in bones and your risk of developing cancer. These three key issues are important to understand if you want to enjoy excellent health during menopause and beyond.

Menopause and your heart

Cardiovascular diseases (CVD) include coronary heart disease (CHD), deep vein thrombosis and stroke. These diseases are among the most common causes of death in both women and men throughout the world, although rates vary from country to country. The rate of occurrence is affected by ethnic background, diet and lifestyle. As with menopausal symptoms, coronary heart disease is more common in countries where the people eat a high-fat diet and have high cholesterol levels.

Women are not considered at risk of CHD until after the age of 55 years, whereas men are at risk at about 45 years. It is believed that the cholesterol in the body changes after menopause, with more total cholesterol, more LDL cholesterol (the bad one) and increased triglycerides. This could increase a woman's risk of developing CVD. How much of this is due to general ageing and how much to decreasing oestrogen is unclear but, whatever the reason, it is very important for women to consider their heart health when thinking about healthy menopause and ageing.

As women suffer more death and disability from CVD than from breast cancer, it is important to understand how our risk increases after menopause and what we can do to minimise it.

Cardiovascular checklist

Tick any of the following that relate to you:

- ❑ Have any of your relatives had CVD?
- ❑ Do you eat a diet high in saturated fats and high in cholesterol?
- ❑ Are you overweight (check the height/weight ratio chart in Step 4, *Exercising for menopause*)?
- ❑ Do you smoke?
- ❑ Have you been diagnosed with high cholesterol?
- ❑ Do you rarely, if ever, exercise?
- ❑ Do you suffer from diabetes mellitus?
- ❑ Do you have high blood pressure?

These risk factors are common to men as well as women for developing CVD. However, there are some risk factors that tend to put women at a higher risk of developing CVD than men, and these include:

- ❑ Are you a diabetic?
- ❑ Do you smoke?
- ❑ Have you been diagnosed with high triglyceride levels and low levels of high-density lipoprotein (HDL)? (You may need to ask your doctor about this.)
- ❑ Are you over 55 years?

As with menopausal symptoms, curious differences in the rates of CVD occur across different cultures. CVD tends to be a predominantly 'Western disease', with women from Westernised countries such as Europe, the United States and Australia having a higher rate than women from developing countries. It is not known to what extent the 'Western lifestyle risk factors' of smoking, high cholesterol, high blood pressure and diabetes have influenced these differences seen across countries.

Research reveals that we need to adopt preventive strategies from the age of 50 years and continue them right through to beyond 70 years to prevent cardiovascular disease. This means making changes now that you can continue throughout your life.

If you tick one or more of the risk factors in the cardiovascular check-list on the opposite page, then you are at a higher risk of developing CVD and will need to take action to reduce that risk as much as possible. If you do not have any of these risk factors, then fabulous! If you put strategies in place now, you have a terrific chance of cutting your risk of CVD. *The Menopause Made Simple Program* has been designed to help you identify strategies to reduce this risk and keep it low for the rest of your life.

The good news is that there are multiple tactics you can use to reduce your risk of both CVD and CHD, including changing your lifestyle. Lifestyle strategies include reviewing your:

- diet
- weight (reducing your weight to the healthy weight range)
- smoking (quitting smoking)
- exercise.

The Menopause Made Simple Program can help you achieve all of these, thereby reducing your risk of cardiovascular disease and ensuring that your heart remains in good shape throughout menopause and well into your future years. You know that you have too much to live for to take this risk. You have no time for heart disease, so why not decrease your risk and give yourself a fighting chance?

Tips for preventing cardiovascular disease

- Modify your diet to make it:
  - low in saturated fat (bad fats)
  - high in good fats (found in fish oils and nuts)
  - low in salt
  - high in fruit and vegetables (variety, seven serves per day)
  - high in phytoestrogens
  - low in cholesterol.
- Ensure that you are the right height/weight ratio (not overweight).
- Stop smoking.
- Undertake cardiovascular exercise (the sort that gets you huffing and puffing) at least five times a week.
- Have your blood pressure and cholesterol checked annually by your doctor.

Menopause and your bones

Osteoporosis is a condition where bones become fragile and may easily break. It occurs more in women than men because of the role that oestrogen plays in bone loss. The rate at which we lose bone differs across the stages of a woman's life.

- Before menopause women have little bone loss.
- After menopause, bone loss increases over the first five to eight years.
- Bone loss continues after menopause and may accelerate again after the age of 75 years.

Women across the world are at different risks of developing fractures. The factors include:

- *Age*. Eighty per cent of hip fractures occur after the age of 75 years.[9]

- *Race.* Western women have the highest rate of osteoporotic fractures, while Asian women have half the fracture rates of Western women.
- *Weight.* Slender women are more likely to incur fractures than heavier women.

Complete the following checklist to identify your risk factors for bone fractures.

Osteoporosis checklist

Tick any of the following that relate to you:

- ❏ Do you have low bone mineral density (BMD)?
- ❏ Have you had a previous fracture?
- ❏ Has your mother had a hip fracture?
- ❏ Are you too light for your weight (underweight)?
- ❏ Do you consume a lot of caffeine (more than the equivalent of three cups of coffee a day)?
- ❏ Do you spend less than four hours a day on your feet? (This risk is increasingly common, with the type of job many of us have.)
- ❏ Are you currently using benzodiazepines or anticonvulsants?
- ❏ Are you unable to rise from a chair without using your arms?
- ❏ Do you have poor depth perception? (You may need to ask your optometrist; it increases your risk of falling.)
- ❏ Do you have poor contrast sensitivity? (Check with your optometrist; this also increases your risk of falling.)

Source: Cummings, 1994

As you can see, a low bone mineral density (BMD) is only one of the risk factors for developing a fracture.

Bone mineral density is a measure of the mass of your bone.

Adding up how many factors you checked in the box is a more accurate predictor of hip fractures than your bone mineral density measurement alone. Whether or not you choose HRT, it is very important to reduce as many of the other factors as possible as the whole aim is to prevent fracturing your bones. Looking at an X-ray of a bone that has osteoporosis, compared with a bone that does not, you can see there is a decrease in bone density—the bone looks thinner. A decrease in bone density gives you a higher likelihood of fracture. The most common bones that fracture are those in your back and the 'long bones'—those in the legs and arms. Fracturing these bones can really affect your ability to get around, so this is an area of your health that you need to take very seriously particularly at menopause and beyond.

In women, the rate of bone loss increases in the five to eight years after menopause, resulting in a loss of about 15 per cent bone loss, then decreases to a much slower pace.

Prevention of osteoporosis

Preventing osteoporosis is an important consideration, to ensure mobility in later years. You need to put preventive measures in place now, whether you are 15, 45 or 60 years old. The earlier you adopt strategies to counteract osteoporosis the better!

- *Family history* and your gene type may be related to your risk of developing osteoporosis. Also, ethnic origin and being female increases the risk.
- Lifestyle factors can increase your risk of bone loss. These include smoking, excess alcohol intake, lack of physical exercise, low calcium intake and inadequate consumption of vitamin D (either from sunlight or your diet).

You can't do anything about your genes, but you can do something about the other factors. Changing these lifestyle factors is part of *The Menopause Made Simple Program*—we show you how to modify these habits to ensure that your bones remain as healthy and strong as possible.

What can you do to decrease your risks?

Strong evidence favours the use of interventions involving diet, exercise and medication if required. Prevention strategies also include increasing peak bone mass, fall prevention, and hormone replacement therapy.

- *Peak bone mass* in women occurs at the age of 25–30 years and is the time of life when you have the most bone mass. Up to the age of 25 years our bones build up this mass, but after that our bone mass starts to decrease. That is why our aim in *The Menopause Made Simple Program* is to increase or maintain the bone mass that you have now so that you stop losing mass or lose it at a slower pace than you might normally.

  Young women should be encouraged and educated to increase their peak bone mass with exercise, calcium and the avoidance of excessive caffeine.

- *Exercise* should be encouraged in both younger and older women. Exercise has been shown to:
  - reverse postmenopausal bone loss, even in women over 70 years of age;
  - reduce the risk of falling;
  - reduce the risk of hip fracture by half;
  - reduce bone loss and back pain in sedentary postmenopausal women.

  The Menopause Made Simple Program includes the third step, *Exercising for menopause*, because it is such an important area in the prevention of osteoporosis, whether or not you choose to take HRT.

- *Fall prevention* involves assessing your environmental hazards. For example, check for slippery surfaces, mats that may be tripped over, or faulty stairs. These checks are inexpensive and have been shown to reduce falls and fractures in older women by half.[10]

- *Hormone replacement therapy.* The main aim for women in relation to osteoporosis is to prevent it from occurring. Many short-term studies have shown that HRT can prevent bone loss.

Tips to prevent osteoporosis

- Undertake weight-bearing exercises (see Step 3).
- Increase your calcium intake to 1500 mg (if not taking HRT) or 1000 mg (if taking HRT).
- Ensure you get adequate vitamin D (get out in the sunshine for ten minutes a day).
- Keep caffeine consumption to a minimum (no more than the equivalent of three cups of coffee per day).
- Watch your weight—if you are too lean (underweight), you are adding another risk factor for developing osteoporosis.
- Check your home and workplace and remove any hazards that may cause you to trip or fall.
- Have your eyes checked to ensure they are in tip-top shape and will not increase your risk of falls.
- If you are constantly sitting down at work, consider going for a walk every two hours around the office. Walk up the stairs, instead of taking the lift. Be creative and find ways to be on your feet for at least four hours a day.

Breast cancer and menopause

Breast cancer is one of the most feared diseases for women. I have been to international conferences where colleagues have asked why women are more fearful of developing breast cancer than heart disease, when there is clearly a greater risk of death from heart disease than from breast cancer.

Is it that women just don't know the facts?

Well, no, it's related to the fact that breast cancer is associated almost exclusively with women and has a much more personal connotation for women than the heart. Women fear the loss of a breast in a deep, inexplicable way.

Breast cancer is the most common malignant disease in women from developed countries (excluding Japan), with the incidence increasing all over the world. As with the rate of hot flushes, there are major differences in the rates of reproductive cancers, including breast cancer and cancer of the uterus, between Western and Asian women.

After 50 years of age, your risk of developing breast cancer increases. Fortunately, you can do a lot to help prevent breast cancer through participation in screening programs.

The two main prevention strategies are having regular mammograms and conducting regular breast self-examinations. The idea of these strategies is to detect any symptoms of breast cancer as early as possible. Early detection improves your treatment choices, your chance of survival and your quality of life with cancer.

Breast self-examination

Breast self-examination is a process of examining your breasts and surrounding areas regularly. It is important that you are aware of how your breasts normally look and feel so that you can detect early any changes that may be due to cancer. By examining your breasts regularly, you may pick up any early symptoms of breast cancer. The changes that you should look for in your breasts and armpits include:

- lumps or lumpiness;
- nipple change—that is, any discharge from the nipple or pulling in of the nipple;
- any change in the shape of the breast or dimpling of the skin;
- an area that feels different from the rest;
- a feeling of pain or discomfort.[11]

Pamphlets on conducting breast self-examination are available from State Cancer Councils and BreastScreen Australia. They explain breast awareness, what is normal and what is not, as well as normal menstrual changes at menopause. It is important to report any changes or findings to your doctor so that they can carry out a professional assessment.

Examine your breasts once a month. Pick a date on the calendar and put a symbol on that date each month to prompt yourself to undertake this very quick but important examination.

Tips for preventing breast cancer

- Conduct regular (monthly) breast examinations and report any suspicious lumps or changes to your doctor.
- Have an annual 'well woman's health check' with your doctor and request a pap smear (to detect cervical cancer), a breast examination and a pelvic examination (to screen for ovarian cancer).
- Undertake regular cardiovascular exercise (see Step 3).
- If you are over 50, have a mammogram every two years.
- Recognise and deal with stress effectively.
- Increase your dietary intake of phytoestrogens and fresh fruit and vegetables (aim for seven serves of fruits and vegetables every day).
- Lower your 'bad' fat intake and increase your intake of 'good' fats (refer to Step 2 to help you change your eating strategies).
- Don't worry—*be happy*!

Mammograms

A mammogram is a screening test which can pick up early cancer of the breast in women. You do not need a referral from a doctor and in Australia mammograms are provided free under the BreastScreen Australia program. Women over 50 years of age are encouraged to have a mammogram every two years. Mammograms are performed by specialist staff trained in breast cancer screening and you will be informed of the results almost immediately.

By undertaking breast self-examination every month and having a mammogram every two years after 50 years of age, you can help to maximise your chances of detecting breast cancer at an early stage.

Summary of Step 1

Menopause is a time of vibrancy and opportunity when you can take control of your life and steer it into the best and most healthful course possible. It is a time for reassessment—this can turn out to be the most positive thing you could do for your body and your life.

Menopause presents an opportunity for you to make changes in the area of preventing cardiovascular disease, osteoporosis and breast cancer. After reading this section, you have the information to realise which symptoms are really associated with menopause and which ones are not. This information can help you make positive changes in your life to ensure that in menopause and beyond you are in peak health in both body and mind.

Q. *I have been feeling really depressed lately and quite suicidal. Is this depression related to menopause? Should I be taking menopausal treatments for it?*

A. No, it is important to recognise that depression is not caused by menopause. Depression is a serious condition that is related to other processes in your body or life at the moment. It needs to be treated appropriately by a qualified health professional.

Q. *I have been experiencing hot flushes and night sweats over the last three months and they are really starting to affect my ability to work and interact with my family. Is there anything that can be done for them?*

A. You have several options which you may like to combine to get the best effect. HRT taken over a short period of time shows excellent results in decreasing hot flushes and night sweats. I would also try increasing your exercise levels. Remember to use paced respiration as you feel the hot flush begin, to minimise your discomfort. The combination of HRT, exercise and paced respirations should have them under control in two to four weeks.

Q. *I am of menopausal age and have had no menopausal symptoms at all. In fact, I feel terrific. Is there something wrong with me? Is there anything that I should be doing?*

A. No, not at all. In fact, many women feel like you! What you can do, however, to ensure that you feel great beyond menopause, is to put in place strategies to minimise your risk of cardiovascular disease, osteoporosis and reproductive cancers.

Step 1

Step 2

Eating for menopause

A healthy eating plan should be adopted throughout life, with a few modifications at different stages of our lives. Eating for menopause is no different. We should eat the foods that provide the body with the best quality fuel available, and enjoy it along the way. It is astounding that healthy eating is often labelled 'boring' eating—usually because of narrow perceptions of what healthy eating involves.

In this step, we look at an eating plan that you can adopt throughout life, no matter what age or sex you are. We then cover the specifics of nutrition that will benefit you before, during and after menopause.

Chapter 6

A healthy eating plan

We are bombarded with information about what is good for us and what we should be eating. A lot of advertising hype surrounds the food we eat, and gimmicky diets make outrageous claims. Use your common sense when delving through this sort of advice. Develop an understanding of how your own body works so that you can make informed decisions. This step will help you to understand the basic principles of nutrition.

Here are four simple guidelines for healthy eating:

- Drink plenty of water.
- Minimise fat.
- Eat a *variety* of fruit, vegetables and wholegrain foods.
- Decrease alcohol, salt and caffeine.

Drink plenty of water

This is a very good place to start healthy eating. To some people drinking water comes naturally, as they have always done so, but for others it may have to be a conscious decision to change a longstanding habit. Many people never reach for a glass of water as a drink on its own. The only way they take water into their body is through drinks such as tea or coffee and sugar-based fluids (soft drinks or cordials). Some foods also contain small amounts of water.

Your body needs water to allow it to function properly, but it's surprising how many people are walking around in a state of semi-dehydration. We are losing water all the time through normal bodily functions and, unless we replace it, the body will run dry.

Aim to drink two litres of water a day—about eight glasses. This may sound a ridiculous amount to some of you, but with a little effort and conscious planning you can easily achieve this on a daily basis. Many women are concerned that if they drink too much water they will be running to the bathroom all the time. At first you will need to go more frequently, but your body will adjust to the increase in fluids over time, particularly as you become fitter. If you are among the one in three women who have a problem controlling their waterworks, you have probably developed a habit of limiting the amount of fluids to minimise the possibility of leakage. In fact, you should be doing the exact opposite—increasing your water intake to retrain your bladder to hold more urine.

Many of the drinks that we count as fluids are in fact diuretics. This means that their effect on the body is to make you lose more water. Caffeine is a strong diuretic and stimulates the body to expel more water. This means tea, coffee and cola-type drinks do not provide your body with the important fluids it needs. In fact, they stimulate the body to lose more water than normal. People who drink a lot of coffee usually don't drink much water and wonder why they feel listless and have a headache at the end of the day. They are dehydrated.

'I don't like the taste of water.' 'Water is tasteless.' These are common responses when we recommend this step to people. The more water you drink, the more your body will crave it. If you particularly don't like the taste of it, use fresh lemon or lime juice to flavour it. Plain sparkling mineral water provides an alternative to still drinking water, and is particularly refreshing with a slice of lemon or lime. Or flavour mineral water with a small amount of fruit juice (try apple or orange, ratio 1:5).

If you are exercising, your body loses more water than usual and this needs to be replaced. Make sure you have a couple of glasses when you have finished your exercise session and sip throughout if available.

Water will also help you lose weight. When you are well hydrated

Tips to increase the amount of water you drink

- Have a jug of water in the fridge at home. Slice some lemon or lime into it if desired.
- Invest in a water bottle to have on your desk at work or at home. Make sure you refill it when it is empty.
- Take a bottle of water out with you and in the car. Sip when you are waiting at traffic lights.
- Have a glass of water when you first wake up.

with water your body functions more effectively in digesting and metabolising your food. Often we mistake thirst for hunger. When the body is dehydrated it may signal us to eat when it really requires water. Water also fills you up so that you don't overeat.

If you are going to change one habit, then this is the one. Drink plenty of water.

Limit your fat intake

We have all heard this before, but what is important is to understand the different types of fat. All fats have the same calorie or kilojoule content, but offer different health benefits to the body. So we should try to minimise the overall amount of fat that we eat, while getting as much benefit as possible from the good fats.

There are three different types of fats: saturated, polyunsaturated and monounsaturated. These terms relate to the chemical structure of the fat.

1. *Saturated fats* are fats that are solid at room temperature and come mainly from animal and dairy products (with the addition of a few plants such as coconut and palm oil).
2. *Monounsaturated fats* are liquid at room temperature. Olive and canola oils, avocados and nuts are all good sources of monounsaturated fats.

3. *Polyunsaturated fats* are also liquid at room temperature. They are contained in most vegetable oils and cold-water fish (salmon, tuna, trout, sardines and mackerel). Some polyunsaturated fats contian high levels of omega 3 fatty acids.

Most foods contain a combination of all three types of fats but in varying proportions. With the low-fat phobia that has been generated, we have confused the fact that there are 'good' fats and 'bad' fats. Good fats consist of monounsaturated fats like olive and canola oil, avocados and nuts. These good fats actually help your body to lower its total cholesterol. Saturated fats are considered bad fats because they contribute to many diet-related health problems.

What is cholesterol?

Cholesterol is required by the body in small amounts for brain, nerve and hormone function. Our body produces the amount that we need, mainly in the liver, and does not rely on cholesterol in the diet. However, the food we eat also contains cholesterol, particularly if it comes from animals—meat, chicken, whole milk, butter and cheese. This means that we usually have too much cholesterol in our bodies.

Cholesterol is made up of LDL cholesterol (low-density lipoprotein) and HDL cholesterol (high-density lipoprotein). LDL cholesterol is commonly referred to as 'bad' cholesterol because it can block arteries. HDL cholesterol is 'good' cholesterol because of its protective effect on the heart.

The different types of fat affect LDL and HDL cholesterol in different ways. Saturated fats, found in foods like fatty meats, chicken, full-fat dairy products, and coconut and palm oil, raise the bad cholesterol (LDL) and lower the good cholesterol (HDL). These saturated fats are also hidden in processed foods such as cakes, biscuits, pies and chocolate. Polyunsaturated fats lower the bad cholesterol. Monounsaturated fats not only lower the bad cholesterol but may also raise the good cholesterol that can help protect the heart.

During menopause—like any other stage of your life—it is important to ensure you keep your cholesterol levels normal. Women entering menopause usually experience an increase in LDL levels and a drop in HDL levels. This means that menopause is a crucial time to ensure that cholesterol levels are controlled. As total blood cholesterol levels increase, so does the risk of coronary disease. Some people are genetically more inclined to high cholesterol levels and need to pay extra attention to keeping them normal. A simple blood test can identify your total cholesterol, as well as your individual readings for HDL and LDL levels. As menopause is a time when the risk of coronary heart disease increases, monitoring your cholesterol levels needs to be routine.

Here are several ways of including good fats in your diet:

- Eat tinned fish (salmon, sardines or tuna in brine or spring water) twice a week.
- Eat a fish meal (preferably deep-sea fish) once or twice a week.
- Use canola margarine spread.
- Use olive oil or canola oil for cooking.
- Make a salad dressing using olive oil, lemon juice and balsamic vinegar.
- Buy breads, muffins, cereals and crackers that contain linseeds.

Omega 3

The omega 3 fatty acids contained in fish, linseed, canola and soy beans have been found to have many beneficial effects on the body, including healthier cardiovascular and immune systems. The food industry has responded to these research findings by producing oils and margarine spreads that contain sources of omega 3 fatty acids.

Omega 3 fatty acids are found in all seafoods. They are particularly high in cold-water fish like salmon, tuna, sardines, trout and mackerel. By including fish in your diet two or three times a week you can ensure you are benefiting from these good fats.

Reducing dietary fat

- *Meats.* Select lean cuts of meat and remove any excess fat and skin before cooking. Avoid or limit processed meats such as sausages, salamis and luncheon style meats.
- *Dairy products.* Substitute low-fat for whole-fat products. These are readily available in most categories. Experiment with different low-fat products in cooking such as natural low-fat yoghurt instead of sour cream, light evaporated skim milk instead of cream. Use light cream cheese instead of butter.
- *Fats and oils.* When cooking use minimal amounts of butter, margarine or oil. Use a cooking spray to decrease the amount used, and non-stick cooking pans. Minimise high-oil dressings.
- *High-fat foods.* Most fast and takeaway foods are high in fat and should be occasional treats only. Cakes, biscuits, chocolate and fried food also fall into this category.

Usually, the more unprocessed a product is the less fat it is likely to contain. A lot of the fat we consume may not be as obvious as the cream in a jam doughnut. That is why it is important to be able to identify the types of foods that are high in fat. By eating mostly natural products, your fat consumption will be automatically reduced.

Many products that we buy have a nutritional label outlining the ingredients and their percentages. It is important to know how to read these labels so you can make informed choices, regardless of what the marketing hype says about a product.

Don't be a sucker. 'Lite', 'low-fat' and 'reduced-fat' are all terms that marketers use to entice us to buy their products. Be careful that you are not drawn to a product solely because of these claims. Read the nutritional labelling to determine exactly how much fat it contains. Sometimes, 'low-fat' foods are not much lower in fat than the original product.

A nutritional information box for baked beans		
	Per 210 g	**Per 100 g**
Energy	840 kj	400 kj
	202 cal	96 cal
Protein	10.3 g	4.9 g
Fat	1.5 g	0.7g
Carbohydrates		
Total	36.1 g	17.2 g
Sugars	9.2 g	4.4 g
Dietary fibre	10.5 g	5.0 g
Sodium	810 mg	385 mg
Potassium	585 mg	280 mg

By looking at the nutritional information box supplied on most pack-
ages you can determine the fat content of the food. You are usually
presented with two columns: one gives the amount of fat per 100 g,
allowing you to compare it with other foods; the second column is the
amount in the recommended serving size.

Eat a variety of fresh fruit, vegetables and wholegrains

This is one of the most important areas of your diet to concentrate on.
The two key words here are *fresh* and *variety*. The fresher the product
the more vitamins and nutrients it will contain. The greater variety of
fruit, vegetables and wholegrains that you eat each day, the more vitamins, minerals and phytochemicals in your diet.

At first this will take a little concentrated effort, because we all get
used to buying the same sorts of foods each week. By trying something
that you wouldn't normally put in your supermarket trolley each week,
you will start to consume a wider range of these products. Start slowly
and introduce changes gradually; over a 12-month period you will have
made considerable adjustments to your diet. Remember, we are looking
at long-term healthy changes to our lifestyle, not quick fixes.

Ideally, aim for seven serves of fruit and vegetables a day. To some people that will seem very high, while for others it is already a daily total. Try to increase the amount of fruit and vegetables you eat to whatever you can manage. This may take time—don't try to change everything all at once.

By increasing your intake of wholegrain products (breads, cereals, pastas and rice) you will increase your complex carbohydrates. Many women feel confused about whether carbohydrates are fattening and tend to steer clear of pasta, bread and potatoes because they are 'starchy'.

Carbohydrates are made up of simple carbohydrates (sugars) and complex carbohydrates (starches). Most sugars (simple carbohydrates) don't add any nutritional value to the diet, only flavour and kilojoules. Exceptions to this are fruit and milk. Both of these contain simple sugars and also other nutritionally important components. Starches— better known as complex carbohydrates—are found in unrefined or unprocessed foods such as vegetables, grains, legumes, nuts, seeds and rice. They are a valuable energy source and assist in regulating blood sugar levels throughout the day (essential for stabilising moods, preventing anxiety and depression). They help to prevent the highs and lows in blood sugar levels that a diet high in simple sugars can cause. Carbohydrates should be one of the main staples of your diet, making up about 60 per cent of your energy value. Complex carbohydrates in their natural state are high in fibre which gives you a feeling of fullness after eating them, requiring less food to satisfy you.

Decrease alcohol, salt and caffeine

You don't need to eliminate these altogether, but moderation is important. Try to keep alcohol consumption to two drinks or less per day and coffee to no more than three cups per day. Salting your food may have become a habit and you will need to train your tastebuds to enjoy food without salt. It is amazing what you can adjust to over time.

Chapter 7

Dietary considerations for menopause

The healthy eating guidelines already discussed in Chapter 6 are important at all stages of your life. During menopause there are certain areas of your diet that need extra focus.

Calcium

We know that calcium is important to our bodies to maintain strong bones, but how many of us are actually getting enough? In our experience very few menopausal women are getting the recommended daily intake (RDI) of 1000 mg per day. If you combine a lack of calcium with the dramatic bone loss that occurs during menopause, then unfortunately fractured bones become likely after the age of 65.

The body cannot produce calcium, so it relies on the amount we take in for important functions involving muscle contractions, nerve impulses and blood clotting. If we do not eat the amount that is required by the body each day, then the body will draw from the stores in our bones. If we are continually lacking in calcium the body has no choice but to deplete these reserves, making our bones weaker each time.

Now is the time to take stock of exactly how much calcium you are getting each day and make adjustments to increase the amount if necessary. You simply cannot afford to overlook this area of your diet.

How much calcium do I need each day?

Women (daily requirements)

Before menopause	After menopause	
1000 mg	Taking HRT	1000 mg
	Not taking HRT	1500 mg

These levels may be higher than some of the recommendations you have seen, but we believe the World Health Organization's guidelines reflect more accurately the amount that is required to maintain optimum health. You will see that the recommendation for women who are not taking HRT is significantly higher (50 per cent more) than women taking HRT. This is an important factor if you choose not to take HRT, as you will need to adjust your diet to reach these calcium levels. Postmenopausal women actually increase their calcium needs as bone loss is accelerated and more calcium is excreted.

To check whether you are getting enough calcium, use the stocktake sheet provided on page 181 and record your diet for three days. This will give you an idea of how much calcium you are getting. It is meant as a guide only and doesn't require you to weigh and measure everything you eat. Simply photocopy the sheet three times, stick it on your fridge and at the end of the day spend a couple of minutes filling it in.

The quantities in the table on page 49 give you an approximate guide of amounts of calcium for a sample day. Use the table on page 50 to work out your average amount for the three days. Compare the amount you are consuming with the recommended intake of 1000 mg if you are taking HRT, or 1500 mg if you are not taking HRT.

If you are not getting enough calcium, work out how much extra you need to consume each day. If you were Cathy in the sample menu plan (on page 49) and you weren't taking HRT, you would need to look at getting about another 500 mg per day. This would be fairly easy to

Cathy's sample menu plan	
Meal	*Approximate calcium content*
Breakfast	
Cup of tea with milk (approx. 50 ml)	75 mg
2 pieces of toast and peanut paste	
Morning tea	
Coffee (no milk)	
Muffin	
Lunch	
Ham and cheese sandwich (25 g of cheese)	250 mg
Banana	
Afternoon snack	
Tea (with milk)	75 mg
Yoghurt	300 mg
Dinner	
Steak and vegetables (carrots, potato, broccoli)	150 mg
Evening snack	
Bowl of ice cream	85 mg
Total (approx.)	1000 mg

do by having cereal with milk in the morning and a glass of milk at some time during the day. This would give Cathy the 500 mg she needed with a little extra to be sure.

You don't have time to work all this stuff out? You really can't afford not to! With the little bit of time and effort it takes to work out your calcium intake you could prevent valuable bone loss over the next 20 to 30 years.

Calcium content

You will see from the table on page 50 that full-fat and low-fat dairy products have the same calcium content. So, even if you are trying to reduce the fat in your diet, you can still ensure that you meet your calcium requirements.

The calcium content of common foods	
Milk (250 ml)	
Full fat, reduced fat, skim	300 mg
Added calcium	440 mg
Soy milk (with added calcium)	300 mg
Cheese	
Cheddar, Edam, Gouda etc. (30 g)	240 mg
Cottage cheese (100 g)	100 mg
Parmesan (40 g)	440 mg
Yoghurt	
Full fat, reduced fat (200 g)	300 mg
Fish	
Canned sardines/salmon with bones (100 g)	300 mg
Fish without bones (100 g)	30 mg
Vegetables (100 g)	
Broccoli, spinach, carrots, cabbage	30 mg
Fruit	
Average 100 g serve	10–30 mg
Orange, medium	30–50 mg
Bread, 2 slices	50 mg
Nuts	
Almonds (30 g)	75 mg
Sesame seeds (1 tablespoon)	100 mg
Egg, 1	30 mg
Tofu (with calcium sulphate) (100 g)	430 mg

Calcium absorption

If you are going to the effort of making sure you get the right amount of calcium, you also want to make sure that your body is absorbing as much as possible. Several factors can assist or inhibit the absorption of calcium in the body.

Vitamin D is important in helping the body to absorb the calcium you consume. Without it the body cannot use the calcium you eat. The body makes vitamin D when our skin is exposed to the sun, and a small amount is contained in foods. With as little as ten minutes of sun per

> **Tips to increase calcium**
>
> - Use calcium-fortified milks. They will give you an extra 140 mg of calcium per every 250 ml glass of milk.
> - Add a tub of yoghurt each day for a morning or afternoon snack.
> - Drink a glass of milk before you go to bed.
> - Include cereal for breakfast a few times per week. You will get about 300 mg of calcium from the milk used.
> - Make a tasty milkshake by blending a banana with skim milk—great for an afternoon snack. Or try other fruits such as strawberries or mangoes.
> - Have a glass of soy milk each day (ensure it has added calcium). The phytoestrogens it contains are as valuable as the calcium.

day, our body can manufacture the amount of vitamin D that it needs. Sunscreen blocks the absorption of vitamin D, so early morning or late afternoon is a good time to get your sunshine quota.

Getting some sun is not a problem for most people, but there are some exceptions. Some elderly people may not have the mobility to go outside or there may be other reasons that prevent them from receiving adequate sunshine. In these situations supplements may be beneficial. Take care that only the correct amount is taken (5–10 mg per day) as excessive amounts can be harmful to the body.

Mother Nature has produced a total package in foods that are high in calcium by including lactose, a natural sugar contained in dairy foods. Lactose enhances the absorption of calcium from these foods.

Excessive caffeine, alcohol and salt will all decrease the amount of calcium you have in your body. Smoking also affects the amount of calcium that is deposited and withdrawn from the bones. If you are a smoker, remember it is never too late to stop. Your body is being affected by this habit at many different levels.

Large amounts of protein (e.g. three large meat meals in one day) will decrease the amount of calcium your body absorbs. This doesn't normally apply to most people. The same applies to excessive fibre in the diet. We all need to ensure that we are getting adequate fibre but not too much—more than 30 g per day usually means that the food will travel through the intestinal gut too quickly and the body won't have enough time to absorb the calcium.

Calcium supplements

Whether you need to take a calcium supplement or not is an individual decision depending on your own circumstances. There is no reason why you can't satisfy all your calcium requirements by eating fresh foods, but if you have reasons that you feel will prevent you getting your daily intake then calcium supplements can be useful. Discuss it with your doctor or dietician to determine the appropriate type and amount.

Dietary supplements should be regarded as just that—'supplements' to your diet. Think of calcium supplements as an addition to your diet where deficiencies occur. If you have determined that you are currently consuming about 600 mg of calcium per day and, for certain reasons, you are not able to increase this amount (e.g. you are intolerant to dairy foods), then a supplement can be beneficial. Use the supplement to make up the difference between what you consume and what you should be having. If you currently get 600 mg per day and recommendations suggest 1500 mg, then a calcium supplement of 1000 mg will provide the difference.

When choosing a calcium supplement look at the amount of elemental calcium that it contains. That is the actual amount of calcium that it supplies.

When we consume calcium through fresh foods, the body receives the amounts spread throughout the whole day. This gives us a chance to absorb maximum amounts of calcium. When we take supplements our bodies are bombarded with one large amount which is not absorbed as efficiently. Try to determine the best time to take the supplement by looking at when you usually get calcium from your food. If you consume large amounts in the morning with cereal or yoghurt, then afternoon or evening might be more beneficial for the supplement.

Phytochemicals and phytoestrogens

Don't let the name fool you—there is nothing new or complex about phytochemicals and phytoestrogens. We have been consuming them since the beginning of time. What we have done recently is to identify their enormous benefit and the contributions they make to our overall health.

Phytochemicals are simply chemicals found in plants ('phyto' means plant). Phytoestrogens are a type of phytochemical. This is the substance that has received so much attention lately, particularly regarding its benefits during menopause.

The important thing about phytoestrogens is that they have a similar structure to the oestrogen we produce in our body. When we consume foods containing these plant oestrogens we can use them in a similar way to the oestrogen we produce. This can be particularly useful when our oestrogen levels decrease during menopause. Nearly all fruit, vegetables and cereals contain phytoestrogens, although the type and amount vary.

There are many different types of phytoestrogens but the most common ones are isoflavones, lignans and coumestans. *Isoflavones* are generally found in legumes, with the highest concentration in soy beans and soy products. *Lignans* are found in most cereals, vegetables and fruits, with high concentrations in oil seeds, especially linseed.[1] *Coumestans* are found in alfalfa and mung bean sprouts, and in red clover.

Combine soy and linseed and you have an excellent source of both isoflavones and lignans, the two phytoestrogens that have been associated with a range of positive health benefits, including reduction of menopausal symptoms. Many soy and linseed products are available, including breads, breakfast cereals and supplements.

Phytoestrogens attracted attention when research studies suggested that people in countries where a diet high in phytoestrogens is consumed have a lower risk of many so-called 'Western diseases'.[2] These include heart disease and cancers such as breast, colon, prostate and uterine cancer.

Sources of phytoestrogens

- *Isoflavones* are found in legumes—these are edible seeds that form within a pod, such as soy beans (including tofu, tempah and miso, which is made from soy beans), chickpeas, lentils, pinto beans, mung beans, kidney beans, peas, lima beans and black-eyed beans.
- *Lignans* are found in linseed; whole grains such as barley, corn millet, oats, rye, rice and wheat; bran, vegetables, legumes and fruit.
- *Coumestans* occur in alfalfa and mung bean sprouts, and in red clover.

Asian countries such as Japan, where they consume large amounts of soy, have much less breast cancer than Western countries like Australia and the United States. However, studies show that when large groups of Japanese women migrate to places such as Hawaii and adopt the local diet, they increase their incidence of breast cancer to reach similar levels to the Americans after a couple of generations. It's suggested that the change from their traditional Japanese diet, which is naturally high in phytoestrogens from miso, tofu and other soy products, to an American-style diet is responsible for the increase in breast cancer.

The benefits of a diet high in phytoestrogens seem to be both short- and long-term for menopausal women.

A study has shown that, in the short term, by increasing the amount of phytoestrogens—particularly isoflavones and lignans—many women experience a decrease in menopausal hot flushes and vaginal dryness.[3] This is good news for women who suffer from the symptoms of menopause, such as hot flushes and a dry vagina—two very common symptoms in Australian women. Perhaps the high levels of phytoestrogens consumed by Japanese women explain the infrequency of flushes and other menopausal symptoms. It's important to note that, in this study, increased daily intakes of phytoestrogens were needed to provide these effects. Also, it was approximately two weeks before any changes in symptoms started to occur and, when the women ceased the increased intake of phytoestrogens, the symptoms of hot flushes and dry vagina returned.

The reduction in hot flushes shown in this study (20–40 per cent) is clearly not as significant as with HRT, but it offers an alternative for women who are unable or unwilling to take HRT.

In the long term, research reveals that phytoestrogens may contribute to the decrease of many lifestyle diseases, such as heart disease, osteoporosis and some hormone-related cancers.

- *Cardiovascular disease.* The lower incidence of cardiovascular disease in Asian cultures and among vegetarians has been linked to the high intake of phytoestrogens consumed by these people. It seems that phytoestrogens have heart-protective qualities. Consumption of soy has been shown to lower total cholesterol levels. Soy not only lowers the 'bad' LDL cholesterol, but also increases the 'good' HDL cholesterol that 'mops up' the cholesterol in the blood. Very few foods have this effect of increasing the good cholesterol in the body.
- *Cancer.* Phytoestrogens may also play a role in decreasing some hormone-related cancers, including cancer of the breast, uterus, colon and prostate. There is a significant difference in breast and endometrial (uterine) cancer between women in Australia and women in Asian countries. Studies strongly support the role that phytoestrogens play in cancer protection—the highest levels of phytoestrogens are found in people living in countries or regions with low cancer rates.[4]
- *Osteoporosis.* The research is scanty in this area, but there is some evidence that isoflavones may help to prevent bone loss. Again, Asian women have fewer hip fractures than Western women and this has been associated with the higher intake of phytoestrogens in their diet.[5]

How much do I need to eat to receive these benefits?

Japanese women can consume up to 200 mg of phytoestrogens per day while most Western diets have as little as 3 mg a day. Women taking 45 mg of isoflavones per day have shown significant beneficial effects. We're not able to make exact recommendations until further studies

---

The benefits of eating more phytoestrogens

Short term

- May decrease hot flushes and vaginal dryness by 20–40 per cent.

Long term

- May contribute to protecting your heart by lowering cholesterol levels.
- May help to combat breast, uterine, prostate and colon cancer.
- May help to preserve healthy bones.

---

have been conducted. Looking at the research to date, the best recommendation seems to be to eat about two soy products per day or four slices of soy and linseed bread (45 mg isoflavones).

Traditionally, Western palates have not been too enthusiastic about the taste of soy. That is why a bread was produced that contained both soy and linseed. This was an easy way for people to include phytoestrogens in their diet without too many changes. By substituting soy and linseed bread for your normal bread, you can get the recommended 45 mg of phytoestrogens per day with four slices.

Many supplements have jumped on the phytoestrogen bandwagon but there is still too little research to determine their value at this stage. Some preliminary studies have produced favourable results with some products (see Step 5, *Alternatives to HRT*). A very important factor is the enormous number of phytoestrogens that are present in foods.

Phytoestrogen values in food

- 300 ml of soy milk contains about 15–20 mg of phytoestrogens.
- 55 g of tofu contains about 35–40 mg of phytoestrogens.
- Four slices of soy and linseed bread contain approximately 45 mg of phytoestrogens.
- 45 g of soy breakfast cereal contains about 36 mg of phytoestrogens.

We really don't understand the interactions between the different phyto-chemicals that occur in foods, so to extract individual phytoestrogens and put them into a tablet form cannot replace a diet high in phytoe-strogens.

Like everything else when it comes to healthy eating, variety is the key. If you can modify your diet to include a range of foods that contain phytoestrogens, then you will be sure of giving your body all the posi-tive health benefits they can provide.

Including phytoestrogens in your daily diet

Breakfast

- Cereal containing soy. Some cereals contain linseeds as well; if not, sprinkle some over the top.
- Two slices of soy and linseed bread with your choice of topping.

Lunch

- Sandwich made with soy and linseed bread; including alfalfa or mung bean sprouts will give you an extra boost of phytoestrogens.

Dinner

- Experiment with dishes containing lentils and soy.
- An excellent cookbook that is full of recipes high in phytoestrogens is the *Natural Alternatives to HRT Cookbook* by Marilyn Glenville.

Snacks

- Soy yoghurt.
- Banana smoothie made with soy milk.
- Fruits, especially apples, citrus fruits, plums and cherries.

If you can add four slices of soy and linseed bread, or a bowl of soy and linseed cereal and a glass of soy milk, per day to the healthy eating prin-ciples we have already discussed (a variety of fresh fruit, vegetables and wholegrains), then you will be getting plenty of phytoestrogens in your daily diet.

Chapter 8

Weight control

Menopause is a time when many women become concerned about putting on weight. Is the weight increase that some women experience due to changing hormones, hormone replacement therapy (HRT) or a change in lifestyle?

Decreasing oestrogen during menopause can change a woman's body from a 'pear' shape to an 'apple' shape. In other words, you move from putting on weight around your hips and thighs to putting it on mainly around your waist. And when we talk about putting on weight, we are really referring to putting on body fat. Excess body fat needs to be produced before it can be deposited somewhere. If your body is not carrying extra body fat then it is not going to be stored, whether on hips and thighs or tummy. The decrease in oestrogen is simply going to alter where the extra fat is stored.

HRT has been blamed for weight gain during menopause, but most studies show otherwise. It seems that weight gain during menopause is more likely to be due to ageing and lifestyle changes than hormones. HRT may cause a bloating feeling in some women, but this is due to fluid retention and not fat, and usually subsides after a short period.

To control weight during menopause the same principles apply as at other stages of your life. The key to maintaining or losing weight is your metabolism. Metabolism is simply how fast or how slowly the body operates. If your body has a high metabolism it is 'idling' fast and therefore using more fuel to function, just like a car. We all know someone who seems able to eat anything but never puts on weight. That is because they have a fast metabolism and their body requires a lot of energy or food to get through the day. Other people seem to have a slower metabolism and put on weight if they even look at food. If this is you, don't despair. There are ways of increasing your metabolism.

- Exercise is crucial to increasing your metabolism and controlling your weight. Strength training is particularly important (see Step 3, *Exercising for menopause*).
- Eat smaller, more frequent meals to keep your metabolism working throughout the day.
- Unprocessed foods, such as fruit and vegetables, require more work by the body to process and therefore keep our metabolism working longer.
- Be more active. Increase your activity throughout the day by taking the stairs, getting up to change the television channel or walking to the shops.

Your body makeup also affects your metabolism. The smaller the amount of muscle mass that you have in your body the lower your metabolism will be. Muscle requires energy from food even when it is not doing anything. If you have greater amounts of muscle in your body and less fat, you will need more fuel or calories each day. That is why men have a faster metabolism than women—they have more muscle mass. As we get older, the metabolism slows down, we are less active and tend to lose some muscle mass. (This is explained in more detail in Step 3, *Exercising for menopause.*)

If you aim to keep your metabolism fast it will help to control your weight.

Diets

Nearly everyone has tried to lose weight at some stage in their life. Currently, about 20 per cent of the adult population are on a diet of some sort. Unfortunately, 99 per cent will fail in their attempt to lose weight and keep it off, because of the simple fact that diets don't work!

Diets don't work because they are a short term solution to a long-term problem. Diets don't change eating habits, which are the cause of the weight gain in the first place. They don't face the problem of metabolism (the 'speed' at which your body functions). Diets actually cause your metabolism to slow down, making weight gain more likely once you resume normal eating. Diets that restrict calories make the body lose lean body mass—that is muscle—together with some body fat. This loss of muscle lowers the body's metabolic rate, which means that fewer calories are used during the day than before. When normal eating resumes, the metabolic rate stays low and the fat returns. You end up with a greater percentage of body fat than before the diet! This is known as the yoyo syndrome.

The only effective means of permanent fat loss is a low-fat eating plan and regular exercise. Nothing else works long term. Slimming diets and appetite suppressants don't work long term. They never have and never will. Neither does liposuction or cellulite creams. They make your wallet lighter but will do nothing for your weight long term.

You will find that exercise and a low-fat diet will benefit you far more than just reducing the waistline. You will feel far healthier, have more energy, be more confident and enjoy life more.

Weight control during menopause

Carrying excess weight is not good for our health at any time but particularly during menopause. Being overweight may also increase our risk of high blood pressure, high cholesterol and diabetes. As the risk of coronary heart disease increases after menopause, we must ensure that we minimise the factors that are going to increase this risk—that is, being overweight.

If you follow the healthy eating principles that we cover in Step 2, one of the benefits you will experience is easier weight control. Put

If you have difficulty losing weight after introducing Step 2's healthy eating principles, then a registered dietician can help you determine where you need to modify your lifestyle.

the emphasis on healthy living instead of losing weight and you will be more successful in maintaining or losing weight. The principles become long-term lifestyle changes instead of temporary weight-loss diets.

Plenty of cookbooks offer healthy low-fat recipes. There are even books available that look specifically at the nutritional needs of menopausal women (i.e. phytoestrogens and calcium). If you are looking for recipe ideas, this kind of book might be where to start. Alternatively, modify your existing diet using the healthy eating principles we have talked about.

Here's a suggested shopping list for the menopausal woman.

- a variety of fresh fruit and vegetables
- low-fat/high-calcium milk
- low-fat soy milk
- soy and linseed bread
- low-fat/high-calcium yoghurt
- breakfast cereal containing soy (with or without linseeds)
- tinned salmon/tuna/sardines
- fresh fish
- raw mixed nuts
- packet of linseeds (sprinkle in muffins or over cereal)
- rice/pasta
- lean red meat/chicken
- olive/canola oil.

These are the basics to add to your shopping list and will obviously vary from person to person. You might add tofu, beans and lentils if you are used to eating them or would like to introduce them into your diet.

We are talking about changing habits. If you can do it for 28 days, you can do it for life.

Food ideas for each meal

Breakfast

We all know that this is one of the most important meals of the day, so if you are not in the habit of having breakfast then start now. If you don't have breakfast your body's metabolism doesn't get kick-started until later in the day. The food you eat for breakfast needs digesting and therefore your metabolism starts working faster. If you have a fast metabolism there is no way your body will let you skip breakfast because you will be too hungry. This will be one of the first signs that your metabolism is getting faster—you will feel more hungry in the early and mid-morning. Vary what you eat each day to ensure you are getting a wide variety of foods.

Some ideas for breakfast include:

- cereal with some sliced fruit (bananas/strawberries)
- toast topped with tomato and avocado
- variety of chopped fresh fruit with natural or flavoured yoghurt
- scrambled eggs—add fresh herbs and a little smoked salmon for a Sunday treat
- boiled/poached egg with toast
- toasted fruit loaf with jam (skip the butter)
- omelette filled with tomato, onion, mushrooms and anything else that takes your fancy
- English muffins with baked beans.

Use a non-stick frypan, so that no or little oil is required. Remember to use low-fat milk and reduce or skip the butter. You won't notice its absence after a while.

Lunch

Lunch doesn't have to be a sandwich every day, although the basic principle of using bread with fillings is a good place to start. We get bored if we have the same thing all the time, but with a little bit of planning and organisation this doesn't have to be the case. Bread comes in all shapes and varieties, so make use of the wonderful array that we have available today. Of course, bread has a limited shelf life but making use of the freezer will enable you to have a variety of breads at hand. Each week, buy a different type of bread to store in the freezer and you will soon have an assortment to choose from.

Try some of these breads:

- pita pockets filled with almost anything you can think of
- flat lavash bread to roll your favourite fillings in
- English muffins are great to top and grill
- mini pizza bread allows you to make a great individual pizza any time of the day
- bread rolls, which come in a variety of types.

Fillings are limited only by your imagination. Use lunchtimes to add extra salad and vegetables to your diet. Fill your bread with lots of these: avocado, tomato, lettuce, mushrooms, carrot, cucumber, sprouts, capsicum and beetroot. Add tuna, salmon, chicken, ham or anything else that takes your fancy. Lunch is an ideal time to add extra fish to your diet by using tinned tuna or salmon a couple of times a week.

Instead of putting these fillings in a sandwich, they can be tossed together to make a salad with a little added dressing. Mix some balsamic vinegar, olive oil and lemon juice for an easy, tasty dressing containing those good fats we talked about. If you are taking lunch to work, put the dressing in a separate container and add just before eating.

Grilling an open sandwich gives different flavour and variety.

During winter, soups are a great means to a nutritious, low-fat lunch that fills you up. Add fresh crusty bread and it will keep you going through the day. Soups are particularly easy to take to work and heat up in the microwave.

Use leftovers from the night before for lunch, if available. Invest in plenty of storage containers to freeze or refrigerate extra helpings. Stir-frys, curries and pastas are great reheated for lunch at work the next day.

Fruit is an excellent way to finish lunch. It is naturally sweet and can take away those sweet cravings you may experience after a meal. Vary the fruits that you eat to ensure you are getting a whole range of goodness. Why not keep a bowl of fruit on your desk. When you do your weekly shopping, buy extra fruit and take it to work. It looks appealing, and you are more likely to reach for the peach if it's in front of you when you feel that 3.30 slump in the afternoon. This will minimise the sweet cravings you get at this time of the day that send you heading for the vending machine or convenience store.

Dinner

Dinner is usually more than just a meal. It is the time of the day when we come together and catch up on the news. Enjoy the food, relax and talk to your family or friends.

Apply the healthy eating guidelines we suggest.

- Include lots of fresh vegetables.
- Minimise the fat. Keep to the good oils, olive oil or canola oil, for the small amount you do use.
- Minimise the alcohol (a daily glass of red wine has been shown to be of benefit in reducing heart disease risk and is also a good source of phytoestrogens).

Try a new recipe at the weekend when you have a little extra time. This will allow you to experiment with new dishes and expand the types of foods you use. Include other family members in the preparation— you will be teaching them valuable skills and it's a great time to talk. Cooking can be made relaxing and enjoyable instead of a chore we dread.

Snacks

Snacks form an important part of the daily diet and a little planning is needed. You may eat three healthy meals a day and then let yourself down by consuming high-calorie/low-nutrition snacks.

Mid-morning and afternoon snacks are a good way to keep your metabolism working throughout the day. They will also keep your hunger under control and prevent bingeing.

Have a variety of snacks and ideas on hand to reach for.

- Yoghurt is a great way to increase your calcium for the day.
- Fruit is the ideal snack, nutritious and portable.
- Dried apricots and raw nuts can be kept in a drawer at work.
- Toasted fruit loaf is tasty and filling.
- Rice crackers with low-fat cream cheese and tomato (some crackers are high in saturated fat, so check the nutritional label).
- Make a batch of low-fat muffins or scones and keep them in the freezer. Microwave one when you feel like a sweet treat.

Take a snack with you if you know you are going to get hungry while out. An apple or banana is easy to put in your bag together with a bottle of water. Remember, we are trying to form new habits—if you repeat it often enough it will become automatic to reach for a piece of fruit and your water bottle as you leave the house or office.

It is important to adopt a balanced approach to healthy eating. Look at establishing long-term healthy eating habits that you can manage and are enjoyable. You don't have to deny yourself anything—a splurge now and then is healthy for the mind.

Jan's story

Jan had battled with her weight for most of her life. Most of the time she was able to keep it under control but recently she found that the kilos were creeping up. In the last five years she had put on 8 kg but Jan put this down to menopause. She was experiencing hot flushes and felt that she had little energy to get through the day. On her last visit to her doctor to have a pap smear he discussed with her the health problems associated with being overweight. Jan's father and sister had died of heart attack and tests revealed her cholesterol was too high. She knew that if she didn't make some changes to her lifestyle she was heading down the same path.

Jan had tried every diet available. She had lost weight with some of

Jan's sample daily eating plan

Breakfast

- soy cereal with low-fat milk (topped with linseeds and sliced fruit)
- cup of tea

Morning tea

- yoghurt
- cup of coffee

Lunch

- sandwich—soy and linseed bread, tuna, tomato, lettuce and alfalfa sprouts
- kiwifruit
- mineral water

Afternoon tea

- smoothie—soy milk and banana

Dinner

- Stir-fry—lean beef strips, loads of vegetables and noodles
- Glass of red wine
- grapes

Supper

- glass of milk
- water throughout the day

them but it always returned when she came off the diet. Jan wanted to feel healthier and decided to change the way she thought about food. Instead of calculating how many calories the food contained, she looked at what foods would help her have a healthier body.

Jan knew she needed to reduce the amount of fat she was eating and have more fruit and vegetables. She started by eating more fruit during the day. This had the effect of cutting down on higher-fat snack foods. Breakfast had always been a piece of toast and a cup of tea, so she introduced variety by eating cereal and sometimes a boiled egg. Jan didn't focus on trying to lose weight, but she did concentrate on eating healthy, nutritious food. Usually, Jan thought of healthy food as boring and tasteless, but as she started to change some of her old eating habits her cravings for sweet and fatty foods decreased.

Jan was aware that calcium is important for women but she had never really been a milk drinker. When she looked at her diet she found that she averaged only one to two servings of calcium a day. She knew that was not enough. Jan introduced a tub of yoghurt each day and started to have a smoothie in the afternoon. She was surprised how she actually enjoyed the taste of the milk when it was mixed with a banana and it filled her up until dinnertime.

Jan replaced her normal bread with soy and linseed bread and started drinking a glass of soy milk each day. After six weeks she felt there was an improvement in the number and severity of her hot flushes.

As Jan realised she had the willpower to improve her diet, she felt confident enough to start doing some walking. She took it slowly at first and walked three times a week. She couldn't believe the difference in the way she felt after just three weeks. After six months Jan knew that she was definitely feeling healthier. She had more energy, was fitter and felt good about life. Another by-product of Jan improving her diet and fitness was that she lost 5 kg.

With a little information, planning and common sense you can enjoy a wonderful array of tasty and nutritious food. Eating a healthy balanced diet is a very important part of the plan we recommend to you for a healthy, manageable menopause.

Summary of Step 2

We have given you a lot of information and suggestions for you to follow to maintain a healthy diet. Let's summarise them.

- Drink plenty of water—aim for two litres a day.
- Minimise fat intake—for the fat you do eat, keep to the 'good' fats.
- Eat a variety of fresh fruit, vegetables and wholegrains.
- Minimise alcohol, salt and caffeine.
- Make sure you get adequate calcium—1000 mg per day if taking HRT, 1500 mg per day if not taking HRT.
- Include phytoestrogens in your diet.

Bon appetit!

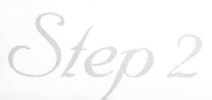

Step 2

Question and answers

Q. *I've heard so much about phytoestrogens and soy and how they can help reduce hot flushes, but I don't like the taste of soy milk. What else can I eat to get the same benefits?*

A. Soy milk is just one of the many foods that contain phytoestrogens. Soy and linseed bread also contains phytoestrogens, as do many soy breakfast cereals. Having a wide range of fresh fruit and vegetables, and a glass of red wine, will also provide your body with the benefits of phytoestrogens.

Q. *I know I should be getting more calcium in my diet but I don't like milk. What else can I eat that will give me enough calcium?*

A. Milk is definitely an excellent source of calcium. You could try disguising the taste in a smoothie made with fruit, yoghurt and milk. Or increase other calcium-rich foods like cheese, yoghurt and fish with edible bones (sardines, salmon). If you find you are not able to get sufficient calcium in your diet then a calcium supplement could be beneficial.

Q. *Since I've been on HRT I've put on 6 kg. I've tried to diet but it just comes back on. I feel as if it's out of control and I don't know what to do.*

A. Many women report weight gain while taking HRT, yet the research suggests this is due more to lifestyle factors than HRT. I'm sure many women would not agree with this, but either way you do have control over the situation. You are not going to lose weight long-term by dieting. You need to take a good hard look at your lifestyle and identify the things that you can change.

Step 2

Exercising is extremely important for losing weight (not to mention the enormous other health benefits you gain).

You need to adopt healthy eating habits for the long term, not diet gimmicks that promise quick fixes. (There is no such thing as permanent quick weight loss; 1–2 kg per month is a good realistic goal.) Healthy eating principles are generally the same for women, men and children.

- Include lots of fresh fruit and vegetables.
- Minimise fat. When you do use fat or oil, keep to the good oils, i.e. olive or canola oil.
- Minimise alcohol, caffeine and salt.
- Drink plenty of water.

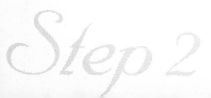

Step **3**

Exercising for menopause

Without a doubt, exercise is the menopausal woman's best friend.

Dr Miriam Stoppard

We all know that we should exercise regularly and we know the reasons why. But are you aware that exercise has a major role in helping you to manage your menopause both physically and emotionally? Even if you have never exercised regularly before, now is the time to start. By exercising, you can minimise the impact of menopause and slow down the ageing process.

In this chapter we look at why exercise can be your best friend during menopause. Weight-bearing exercise (together with adequate calcium) will help you not only *maintain strong bones*, but *strengthen the muscles* that help you keep your balance and mobility. This is a crucial factor with ageing—the old saying 'Use it or lose it' is true. The less we move, the weaker we get because our muscles are not being made to work and our bones become less dense and brittle. Also, weight gain can be a real concern for many women during and after menopause. The key to maintaining our weight at any age, but particularly as we get older, is exercise.

The type of exercise you choose during menopause is important, and we explain the different types of exercise you need to include to maximise the benefits. We outline the easiest way to achieve your goals by looking at *what type of exercise*, and *how much* and *how hard* you need to exercise.

It's no good knowing all the right facts if there is no action. We help you to overcome the main obstacles that women experience with exercise and explain how to design a realistic and achievable exercise program.

9

The benefits of exercise

You will experience many physical and emotional benefits when you exercise regularly. Exercise will:

- maintain strong bones
- strengthen your muscles
- keep your balance
- help you maintain your weight
- minimise lifestyle diseases
- increase your confidence and self-esteem.

Exercise maintains strong bones

We tend to take our bones for granted, without giving them much thought, until we break one of them and realise the all important function they play in supporting us through everyday life. We think of our bones as dormant parts of our body, not really experiencing many changes, unlike our muscles, heart and lungs. However, the situation is quite the contrary. Bones are living structures that are changing all the time.

It's important to have a general idea of how our bones work in order to understand the enormous benefits of exercising. As well as holding us up and protecting our organs, bones are where we store calcium in the body. They act like a bank, where we can make deposits of calcium and withdrawals when we need them. To allow the calcium to move into and out of the bone there are special bank tellers (or cells) that are responsible for this. There are two types of cells—osteoblasts and osteoclasts. The osteoblasts make all the deposits of calcium into the bones. The osteoclasts withdraw or break down calcium from our bones when we need it in other places such as nerves or muscles, or for blood clotting. These deposits and withdrawals continue all the time.

As with any bank account, the more deposits you put in the healthier it looks. If you were to continually withdraw from your account without making many deposits, you would soon be in the red. The same applies to your bones. The body withdraws calcium from the bones continuously and if we are not making sufficient deposits of calcium we soon have bones that are less dense and more susceptible to fractures. This can lead to a condition called *osteoporosis*.

Osteoporosis

As you can see from the life cycle of the bone, we start to lose the density of our bones as we get older. The lower the bone density, the weaker the bones become. Osteopenia is the process of declining bone density, with osteoporosis the next stage. Osteoporosis is a disease that works silently in the body; usually a fracture is the first sign.

Life cycle of a bone

0–20 years	You lay down more bone than you lose.
20–30 years	Bone density is maintained: the amount you use equals the amount you lay down.
30–menopause	The scales start to tip and you begin to lose bone.
First 5 years after menopause	Critical time—preventive measures must be put into place to minimise bone loss.
55–70 years	Bone loss slows down.
70+ years	Bone loss slows down still further.

When our bones lose density they become brittle because the internal structures have weakened. A normal healthy bone looks like honeycomb inside, whereas an osteoporotic bone looks more like swiss cheese, with large holes of air that don't give much support to the bone structure.

Menopause is a critical time for bone loss because the decrease in oestrogen slows down the formation of bone. If preventive measures are not put into place, women can lose up to 1–2 per cent of bone density per year. If this bone loss is allowed to continue into later years, osteoporosis may be the end result.

Like most diseases, there are certain risk factors that will increase your chances of getting osteoporosis. But there are many that you can control by making simple adjustments to your lifestyle.

Go through the checklist below and tick the boxes that apply to you.

Can't change
- ❏ I am female
- ❏ I am menopausal age or over
- ❏ My mother or grandmother had osteoporosis
- ❏ I have a thin/small-framed body
- ❏ I am Caucasian or Asian

Can change
- ❏ I have a poor diet (particularly lack of calcium)
- ❏ I have low physical activity
- ❏ I smoke
- ❏ I have two or more alcoholic drinks per day
- ❏ I have more than four cups of coffee per day

The more boxes you ticked, the greater your chance of developing osteoporosis at some stage of your life. If you have ticked any factors in the 'Can change' category, now is the time to do something about them.

Calcium and exercise

The good news is that you can help to build up and maintain healthy deposits of calcium in your bones by having adequate calcium in your diet and taking regular exercise. We discussed the importance of calcium in Chapter 8. Now we look at exercise and the best type for you to do.

Any exercise is better than nothing, and that's an important thing to keep in mind. Just start moving about more—that's the first step.

But some exercises will definitely give you more benefits than others when it comes to maintaining strong bones. Weight-bearing exercise is what we need to focus on when choosing the type of exercise we're going to do. Weight-bearing exercise refers to any exercise where you support your own body weight during the activity, usually done in an upright position.

When we do weight-bearing exercise the force of gravity puts beneficial stress on our bones. This stress is caused by the pull from the muscles attached to the bone. When these muscles are worked in a way that is different from everyday activity it stimulates the formation of new bone.

Weight-bearing activities
- walking
- dancing
- running
- aerobics
- strength training
- tennis
- golf.

Non-weight-bearing activities
- swimming
- cycling
- aqua-aerobics.

Even though water-based activities have less benefit in maintaining strong bones, when combined with weight-bearing exercise they provide many other positives.

Exercise strengthens the muscles

Loss of muscle strength was once thought to be part of the ageing process. Research now proves that this loss of muscle strength can not only be delayed but reversed. The main reason we start to lose strength as we get older is because we are losing muscle mass. Muscle mass is the amount of muscle we have in our body. This loss of muscle mass is not one of the results of ageing—it is caused by the decrease in activity that occurs as we get older. It is quite different from the loss of bone we experience. Bone loss will happen, no matter what we do. We can only minimise it.

Loss of muscle is a different ball game—it occurs simply because we slow down and do less. It then becomes a bit of a cycle: the less we do, the more muscle we lose, the less we are able to do. The term 'Use it or lose' is so true. If you don't use your muscles you will lose muscle mass and consequently strength. The first astronauts experienced the dramatic effects of muscle loss in space. Because they didn't use their muscles in the weightless environment they experienced significant muscle loss and strength in just a few days.

Why strength is important

As we start to lose strength we find everyday activities harder to do. This creeps up on us, until one day we admit that something we have always been able to do without thinking about it has become difficult (e.g. carrying wet clothes and hanging them on the clothes line or taking shopping bags in from the car). Our muscles move us around all day, performing tasks, and the stronger they are the more easily we can do these activities.

Without adequate muscle strength we begin to lose our balance and mobility. As muscle mass decreases, our balance becomes poorer. They go hand in hand. As our balance declines we begin to lose confidence in some activities and modify our lifestyle. Again the cycle continues.

Being strong can actually help you maintain or lose weight as you get older. Strength is directly related to the amount of muscle mass you have—the stronger you are, the more muscle mass you have. An increase in the amount of muscle also increases your metabolism.

The key to maintaining our weight at any age, but particularly as we get older, is to keep our metabolism high. Our body composition (i.e. how much muscle and fat we are made up of) determines the speed of our metabolism. Muscle is an active tissue and uses energy to function; stored fat is mostly inert and requires no fuel. As we get older we are less active and therefore lose muscle. The more body fat and the less muscle we have, the slower the body operates. Regular exercise, especially strength-training activities, will keep your metabolism high and help control weight gain.

Exercise for strength

When we do certain exercise (i.e. strength-training exercise) our body responds by becoming stronger. This occurs because the extra load that our muscles have to lift causes minute tears in the muscle fibres. Don't be alarmed when I say this, because this process is very beneficial to our bodies. Our muscles respond to these forces by becoming stronger and slightly larger.

Strength or weight training is by far the most effective way of maintaining and improving our strength. This is usually done by performing particular exercises with a weight or machine. You make the muscle work harder than it is used to and it responds by getting stronger.

It is clear from all our time working with women and exercise that this is the main area that is not understood.

'I'll become big and bulky'

This is usually the first thing women say to me when I recommend strength training as part of their exercise program. It is a myth. I cannot stress enough that strength training exercise is one of the most beneficial activities you can incorporate into your healthy lifestyle plan. It won't make you bulky—in fact the opposite is true. Muscles become more toned, giving a leaner, more defined look. The muscle-bound body builders that we usually associate with strength training achieve this look from hours upon hours every day of lifting incredibly heavy weights. This is not what we are suggesting for you.

Exercise helps to maintain balance

We tend to take the ability to balance for granted until we start to lose it. After the age of 40 our balance starts to decline. At first these changes are so small we don't notice them. But if nothing is done to combat these changes, we'll become very aware of a decrease in balance in our seventies and eighties. About 30 per cent of people over the age of 65 report at least one fall a year. If bones are weak due to osteoporosis this fall can be devastating, with fractures to the hip, back or arms.

The decline in balance as we get older is directly related to the decrease in muscle strength due to inactivity. So, when we increase our strength through exercise we are also improving our balance. The decline in ability to balance as we get older is gradual and may go unnoticed because moving and walking are adjusted to compensate for it. If you watch older men and women walk, they often have their feet wider apart to give them a bigger base of support on the ground. They tend to shuffle, because not lifting their feet high gives them a more stable feeling. These adjustments to their gait are usually subconscious and happen over a long period of time.

All too often we believe that these changes are out of our control. Exercise allows you to prevent or minimise this loss of balance. You can ensure that you walk with confidence now and into your older years.

Exercise helps to maintain weight

Maintaining their weight is usually a big concern for women during menopause. Many women say they are more prone to gain weight and tend to put it on more around the stomach. Exercise is absolutely crucial during this time to enable women to manage their weight.

The decrease in oestrogen affects where you are more likely to increase weight. Premenopause, women tend to put on weight around their hips and thighs. It is that little reserve that Mother Nature gives us to ensure enough food for our unborn children. During and after menopause, when oestrogen supplies are decreased, extra fat is stored around the tummy area, similar to men. We move from the pear-shaped body to more of an apple-shaped body. Unfortunately, storing body fat around the mid-section is far more dangerous to our health. Fat can accumulate around our vital organs, especially the heart, leading to heart problems, so it is very important that we don't let our weight get out of control during this period.

Exercise is one of the key factors in weight control. It is very difficult to lose weight and keep it off long term if you are not exercising regularly. Exercise helps to keep your metabolism high, which means your body will burn more calories in everything it does (even when you are sleeping). And the more muscle you have in your body the higher your metabolism. Combine this with the extra energy you burn up when you exercise and you will find your weight easier to maintain.

Exercise minimises lifestyle diseases

In most Western countries there has been a dramatic increase in a range of diseases associated with our modern lifestyle. These include:

- cardiovascular disease
- high blood pressure and cholesterol
- adult-onset diabetes.

They are called lifestyle diseases because they are affected by aspects of our lifestyle, such as diet, activity and exercise levels and stress. By controlling your weight, exercising regularly and keeping stress levels under control, you can minimise your chances of developing these diseases, or keep them at a manageable level. The incidence of these lifestyle diseases increases as we get older, so menopause is a very important time to put these preventive steps into place.

Cardiovascular disease

Cardiovascular disease refers to health issues connected with the heart (cardio) and associated arteries and veins (vascular). Whether you are going to have problems with cardiovascular disease is determined by three main factors:

1. *Your family history* of cardiovascular disease: have your mother, father, grandparents, brothers or sisters had problems with their heart?
2. *Lifestyle*—diet, exercise and stress.
3. *Age*—the older you are the higher the chance of cardiovascular disease.

Before menopause, women have a lower risk of cardiovascular disease than men, but as they get older this difference disappears. Menopause is thus a very important time to ensure that you are doing all you can to minimise your chances, especially if you have a family history of heart disease.

High blood pressure and cholesterol

Both blood pressure and cholesterol levels are affected by the same risk factors as cardiovascular disease—family history, lifestyle and age. If high blood pressure and/or raised cholesterol levels are not controlled they can lead to cardiovascular problems.

Diabetes (type 2 adult-onset diabetes)

There are two types of diabetes: type 1 (juvenile-onset diabetes) and type 2 (adult-onset diabetes). Type 1 occurs in childhood and has to be controlled by insulin injections throughout life. Type 2 diabetes occurs in adults and is usually related to being overweight due to the type and quantity of food consumed. Ninety-five per cent of all diabetes is adult-onset diabetes. In type 2 diabetes, losing weight and improving the diet (including more complex carbohydrates and reducing sugar and fats) is usually successful in improving the problem.

To improve your diet, follow the healthy eating principles outlined in Chapter 8:

- Drink plenty of water.
- Minimise fat intake (and stick to the 'good' fats).
- Eat a variety of fresh fruit, vegetables and wholegrains.
- Decrease caffeine, salt and alcohol (one glass of red wine per day is beneficial).

Keep active and do cardiovascular or aerobic exercise three to five times per week. This type of exercise will help keep your heart strong and your blood pressure and cholesterol at normal levels. We discuss cardiovascular and aerobic exercise more fully in Chapter 10.

Don't let stress take over your life. A certain level of stress is normal and allows us to function effectively. But if we are continually stressed our bodies are affected by the constant stimulation of the brain. You need to be aware of what works for you and identify when too much stress is affecting you. Introduce strategies that enable you to control the stress in your life.

- Exercise regularly.
- Have some personal relaxation time.
- Maintain interests and hobbies outside work.
- Adopt a positive mental attitude.
- Be organised, prioritise and plan your day.
- Look after yourself. Get plenty of sleep, eat well and enjoy a little self-pampering!

Exercise increases confidence and self-esteem

We have talked about the enormous physical benefits associated with exercise, but we cannot overestimate the increase in emotional well-being at the same time. So many of these aspects are interrelated that it is difficult to single them out individually. It becomes a cycle where the physical and emotional benefits are intertwined. As you become fitter and healthier, your self-esteem improves and you continue to exercise and make healthy food choices, and this makes you feel more confident. Thus the cycle continues. Unfortunately, this cycle also works in reverse. The less active you are, the less you want to do, the more you eat, the lower your self-esteem, and so on and so on.

Exercise lifts depression and helps combat sluggishness, which makes weight management easier. When we exercise, our body releases a hormone called endorphins. This is a natural 'feel good' drug that gives us a 'high' after exercise. There is no easier way to achieve that 'get up and go' feeling that we all crave.

Chapter 10

Choosing your exercise

*The body is... our vehicle for being, for loving, for moving, for feeling—
and if it doesn't work, it's fairly certain nothing else will work either.*
                                                    Diana K. Roesch

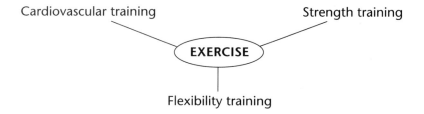

There are many different types of exercises that you can do and some
will give you more benefits than others. But start with something
you enjoy—anything is better than nothing.

Our theory is that if you are going to exercise you might as well get
the most out of it. So we are going to recommend the ideal exercise
program for the menopausal woman. This includes cardiovascular,
strength and flexibility training.

Cardiovascular exercise

Cardiovascular, or aerobic, exercise is any exercise where you feel your heart rate increase. As you walk, run, swim, cycle or dance, the blood starts circulating faster and your heart beats more quickly. Your heart is made of muscle and, like any other muscle, as it is worked harder it gets stronger. The stronger your heart is, the healthier it is. Aerobic exercise, therefore, is very important in decreasing lifestyle diseases.

Without a doubt, the easiest form of aerobic exercise is walking. Walking has the added benefit of being weight-bearing as well as aerobic. You can start slowly and build up gradually. It doesn't have to be expensive—you need little equipment other than a comfortable pair of walking shoes. The benefits of a simple 30-minute walk three to five times a week are amazing. It can decrease your risk of heart attack, lower your chances of osteoporosis and help reduce your weight.

Aerobic exercise
- walking
- swimming
- running
- cycling
- aerobic classes
- dancing
- some exercise machines (e.g. stair climbers, treadmills)
- tennis (depending on the level).

Non-aerobic exercise
- yoga
- weight training
- tai chi
- lawn bowls
- golf.

Walking

Start off by choosing a comfortable pair of walking shoes. They don't have to be the latest design or cost a fortune. Always wear cotton socks so your feet can breathe. If you go to buy a pair of shoes, take the socks that you will wear to try them on. Replace your shoes when they start to get worn, probably every six months.

If you haven't walked for a long time, start slowly and increase the distance as you begin to feel fitter. Believe it or not, that will happen more quickly than you think. The rule of thumb is: you should still be able to hold a conversation with someone throughout the walk. If you can break into a song, then speed it up a bit.

- When you walk, think tall. Eyes should look forward not at the ground. Your shoulders and back should be relaxed, arms slightly bent and swinging naturally. (Don't worry about getting the power-walking arms.)
- Think about tightening your stomach muscles slightly with your back straight.
- Don't carry weights. They are not going to tone your arms, and put unnecessary stress on your shoulders and neck.

When you start walking, keep the pace slow for the first five minutes to allow your muscles to warm up. Then increase to your comfortable walking pace for 20 minutes, slowing down the pace for the last five minutes to cool down. I suggest stretching at the end of the walk, as it doesn't break your pace and your muscles are warm (see stretches on page 100).

You could start with a five or ten minute walk and build up to 30 minutes over a period of four weeks. Remember: the key with exercise is to start slowly and build up gradually. Consistency pays off.

No matter what cardiovascular or aerobic exercise you decide to do, aim to build up to 30–45 minutes per session. It might take you eight weeks to achieve this aim. Start slowly and build up gradually. If you can manage three to five cardiovascular sessions a week, you're doing well.

Strength training

Strength training may be quite foreign to you and may cause you anxiety initially. But please persevere with it. The benefits you will receive from just two sessions a week are enormous. These include significant increase in muscle strength, bone density and balance, not to mention a trimmer, toned body shape.

You will need some guidance with this area. You could follow the exercises outlined in this book or engage a fitness trainer. If you decide to try these exercises at home, here are a few things to think about.

- Choose a time of the day that is going to suit you best.
- Wear comfortable clothes.
- Select a place where you have room to move. It doesn't have to be very large, as long as you can lie down. Have a mat or soft towel to lie on when doing floor exercises.
- Remember: start *slowly* and build up *gradually*.

If doing the strength exercises at home, start with Program 1 exercises that do not use dumbbells. These don't involve any money outlay, just your time and motivation.

Program 1   Exercises (no equipment)

- squats
- lunges
- modified pushups
- seated tricep dips
- abdominals and pelvic floor
- lower back
- stretches.

Use the pictures and descriptions to guide you through the program. (The stretches are shown on pages 100–1.)

'Reps' and 'sets'?

A 'rep' refers to a repetition of an exercise. Each time you perform the exercise it is one repetition or 'rep'. A 'set' is made up of a group of repetitions. Here, you will be doing two sets of 8–10 reps.

When we talk about 8–10 repetitions we want you to do a minimum of eight and a maximum of ten repetitions. If you can't do eight repetitions of the exercise then the weight is too heavy and you need to move to the lighter weight. If you can do more than ten repetitions, the weight is too light and you need to move to the next heavier weight.

You will find that the weight you start with will grow too light and you will be able to perform ten reps easily. That is the time to move to a heavier weight. If you don't increase the weights when they get too light, your muscles will not continue to get stronger. This increase in weight will be different for each exercise. Some you will increase more quickly than others. This is perfectly normal.

Squats

This is an excellent exercise that will help strengthen your leg and bottom muscles.

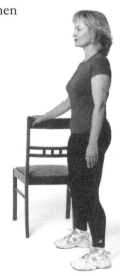

- Use a chair to start with. This will give you support and help you keep your balance. Pick a chair that is sturdy and high enough to lean on comfortably. You should just be lightly touching the back of the chair, not gripping tightly.
- Place feet shoulder width apart.
- Eyes looking forward, to help keep your back straight. If you look down at the ground, your back will hunch over.
- Bend your knees, lowering your body as though you were going to sit on a chair.

- Raise your arms forward (only one if you are using the chair).
- Hold for one second, then rise to a standing position. Don't lock your knees in when you stand up—keep them slightly bent and 'soft'.
- Give yourself three seconds rest between each repetition (rep).
- Do 8–10 repetitions, then repeat the set. Give yourself 1–1½ minutes rest between each set to allow your muscles to relax.
- You can adjust the difficulty of the exercise by varying how far you squat down. When starting off, lower your body a short distance and slowly build up to full squat. You should never go lower than a 90-degree angle of your knee.
- When you feel comfortable, try performing the exercise without the chair.
- If you feel discomfort in your knees, don't go down as far until your leg muscles strengthen.

Lunges

Lunges not only strengthen the legs, but also help to tighten and lift the bottom.
- Use the chair initially to keep your balance, fingers resting lightly on the backrest.
- Start with feet together and take a large step forward. This will lower your body down. Hold for one second and return to a standing position with feet together.
- Step forward with your opposite foot and repeat.

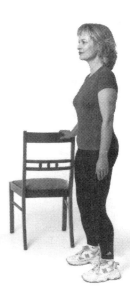

- Make sure you are stepping far enough forward so that your foot is in front of your knee as you bend down.
- Keep your eyes looking forward, not down. Keep your back straight.
- Start with ten repetitions, five on each leg. Increase to two sets of 8–10 repetitions on each leg.
- As with squats, if your knees give you discomfort lower yourself only slightly.

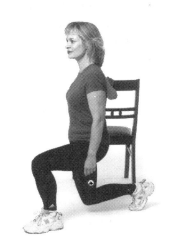

Modified pushups

Pushups are a great exercise to strengthen your upper body without using weights. You use your body as a resistance instead of a dumbbell. There are two levels of modified pushups. Start with level 1 and progress to level 2 when you feel comfortable.

Level 1

- Use a mat, rug or towel to provide some cushioning for your knees.
- Get down on 'all fours' on the floor.
- Hands should be shoulder width apart, with fingers pointing forward.
- Bend at the elbows to lower your chest and head towards the ground.
- Bottom should be sticking up in the air.

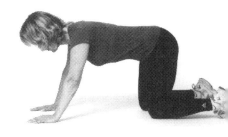

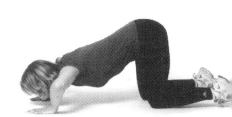

- Hold for one second, then straighten your arms to raise the body back to the original position.
- Think about tucking in your tummy and keeping your back flat.
- Do two sets of 8–10 repetitions.
- Don't tense neck and shoulders; relax as much as you can throughout the exercise.

Level 2

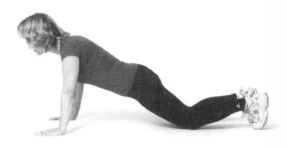

- Start with your knees on the ground as in level 1 but tuck your bottom in to form a straight line from shoulders to knees. Place your hands, palms down, to the side of your shoulders, fingers facing forward and elbows slightly bent.
- Bend your elbows to lower your chest towards the ground. Stop just before your body touches the ground and hold for one second.

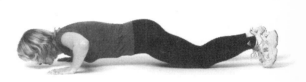

- Return to the starting position.
- Think about tucking in your tummy and keeping the body straight.
- Pause for one second, then lower your body to the starting position.
- Do two sets of 8–10 repetitions.
- Make sure you don't hold your breath. Your breathing will adjust to a natural rhythm as you perform the exercise.

Seated tricep dips

This exercise strengthens the triceps, the group of muscles at the back of the arms. If you hold your arms out straight, it is the 'bat wing' area that women complain of. There are two levels. Start with level 1.

Level 1

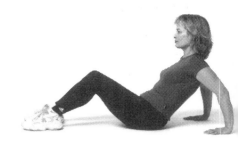

- Sit on the ground with your knees bent and feet flat on the ground. Put your hands on the ground behind you slightly wider than your shoulders with your fingers pointing towards your bottom.
- Straighten your arms until your elbows are 'soft'.
- Keep your bottom on the ground and bend your elbows to lower your body.

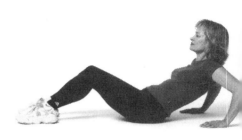

- Hold for one second, then raise to starting position.
- Keep your tummy tucked in and shoulders back.
- Do two sets of 8–10 repetitions.

Level 2

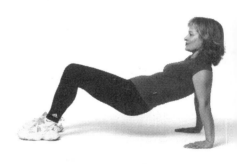

- Start in the same position as level 1.
- As you straighten your arms, lift your bottom off the ground.
- Hold for one second, then lower to the ground. Stop just before your bottom touches the ground.
- It is important to make your arms do the work. Don't bounce up and down using your legs. Your body should move only because you are bending or straightening your arms.
- Do two sets of 8–10 repetitions.

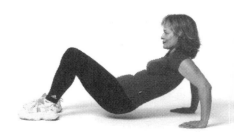

Abdominals

Everyone I have ever worked with is keen to 'tighten' their stomach. Having strong abdominals will help support your body and take the strain off your back.

BRACING THE ABDOMINALS

When you perform abdominal and pelvic floor exercises it is important to stabilse or 'brace' the abdominals to give maximum support.

- Lie on the ground on your back with knees bent and head relaxed down.
- Put your hands on your hips with fingers touching the groove of the groin area. Suck in your lower abdominals and hold. You should feel the area near your fingertips tighten. The area of your upper abdominals should remain relaxed.
- You should be able to breathe normally as you keep them contracted.
- It may take a bit of practice to get this one right, but persevere.

The bracing of the abdominals should be done at the start of all your exercises.

ABDOMINAL CURLUPS

- Lie on the ground on your back, on a mat or towel. Knees should be bent and feet flat on the ground.
- Rest your hands on your thighs.
- Brace your abdominals and hold.
- Lift your head and shoulders off the ground and slide your hands up towards your knees.

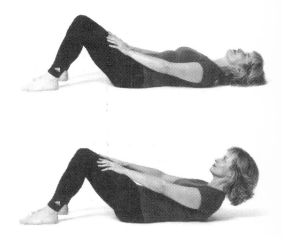

- Hold for one second, then return to the starting position.
- Keep shoulders and neck relaxed as much as possible. Tuck in your chin slightly.
- Wait for three seconds, then repeat.
- Do two sets of ten repetitions. (Build up to 20 as you get stronger.)
- You should feel your abdominals contracting; if you touch them lightly as you lift, they will feel harder.
- As you get stronger, lift your hands up higher towards your knees. You are not aiming to lift your body fully of the ground. That would put too much strain on your back.

If you feel discomfort in your neck, you need to try to relax your neck and shoulders. You might find it easier to support your neck by putting your hands behind your neck. Interlock your fingers to provide a 'cushion' for your neck to rest in and think about your head relaxing on a 'pillow'. It is important not to pull on your neck with your hands.

Abdominal curling machine

There is a lot of abdominal exercise equipment that helps to support your neck as you lift. Most of this equipment is fairly safe, depending on the angle of the head-rest. If you have one of these gathering dust in the garage, pull it out and try doing the abdominal curlup exercise with it. You might find it more comfortable with your neck supported, or you might find it more natural without. Choose what is most comfortable for you.

Pelvic muscle exercises

While you are in the lying position, perform the pelvic muscle exercise plan on page 106. We discuss pelvic floor muscles and the role they play in Chapter 11.

Lower back

The lower back needs strengthening just like any other muscle. The alternate arm and leg raise is suitable for people with lower back problems. In fact, it is even more important for those who have problems with the lower back.

- Lie on your stomach with both hands stretched out straight above your head.

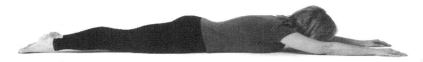

- Lift up your right arm and left leg at the same time.
- Hold for one second and relax.

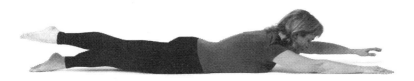

- Repeat with the left arm and right leg.
- Do two sets of 8–10 repetitions.
- Don't lift your arms and legs too high. Aim for about 10 cm off the ground.

When you have been doing Program 1 for six weeks, you might like to invest in some dumbbells that will allow you to work that little bit harder (Program 2).

Initially, look at purchasing one pair each of 2-kg, 3-kg and 4-kg dumbbells. Any fitness equipment supply store will stock these.

As with any strength-training exercises, when using dumbbells it is important to think about the way you are doing the exercise. Follow the pictures we provide and concentrate on moving in a *slow* and *controlled* way. Technique is important.

Program 2   Exercises with dumbbells

- squats
- lunges
- modified pushups
- shoulder press
- tricep extension
- abdominals and pelvic floor
- lower back
- stretches.

Some of these exercises are the same as in Program 1.

Squats

Use the same technique as in Program 1 but add some dumbbells. Start with 2 kg in each hand and increase the weight as you feel it becoming too light.

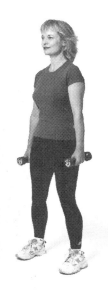
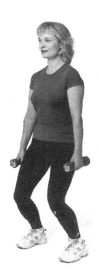

Lunges

Take a 2-kg weight in each hand and perform the same exercise as in Program 1.

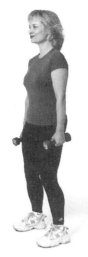 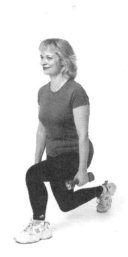

Modified pushups

As in Program 1. Try level 2 if you feel you can handle it.

Shoulder press

This exercise will work the muscles of your shoulders.

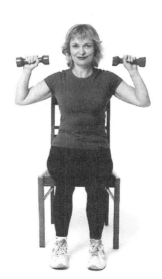

- Sit in the chair with your back straight. Tighten and brace the abdominals. Keep them tucked in throughout the exercise.
- Start with the dumbbells pointing to the side, level with your shoulders.

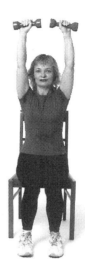

- Straighten your arms above your head so that the dumbbells meet.
- If you can't see the dumbbells above your head, they are too far back. Bring them slightly forward.
- Bend elbows and lower dumbbells to shoulder height.
- Do two sets of 8–10 repetitions.

The following two exercises work your arm muscles. Triceps are at the back of the arms and biceps are at the front.

Bicep curl

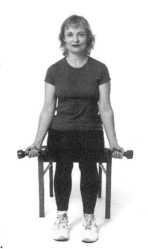
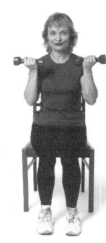

- Sit in the chair with your back straight, abdominals tucked in and braced.
- With a dumbbell in each hand, start with the arms straight by your side, close to the hips.
- Lift both hands together to bring the dumbbells up to your shoulders.
- Hold for one second.
- Slowly lower the weights down to the starting position. (Don't let them fall down.)
- Do two sets of 8–10 repetitions.

Overhead tricep extension

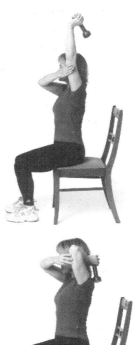

- Sit on the chair, back straight, abdominals tucked in and braced.
- With a dumbbell in your right hand, start with it straight above your head. Place the other hand on the elbow of your straight arm to give it support.
- Bend elbow so the dumbbell is lowered to the back of your shoulder.
- Straighten arm and lift dumbbell to the starting position.
- Don't let the arm fall forward throughout the exercise. Use the opposite arm to support and keep it back in position, especially as you start to get tired.
- You should be feeling this in the back of the arm.
- Do two sets of 8–10 repetitions.

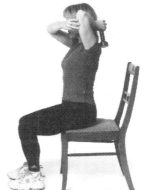

The rest of the exercises—abdominals, pelvic floor, lower back and stretching—are the same as in Program 1.

If you decide to go to a fitness centre, they will probably provide you with an individual program. A fitness centre will have a range of machines and equipment to strengthen different muscles. A fitness instructor will show you how to do the exercises and how to use the equipment.

Program 3 is a program you can follow in a fitness centre, using their equipment.

Program 3   Exercises in fitness centre

- squats
- lunges
- chest press (machine)
- lateral pulldown (machine)
- shoulder press
- tricep extension
- abdominals and pelvic floor
- lower back.

A fitness centre should have equipment to perform all of these exercises and a fitness instructor will be able to modify any exercises to accommodate specific equipment.

Stretching/flexibility

Flexibility is one of the most underrated types of fitness. Stretching is important to help minimise injuries and to allow your muscles and joints to perform their best range of movement. Stretching can be done as part of a cardiovascular or strength exercise session, or separately, in a yoga class for instance. To get the most out of stretches, the muscles should be warmed up. As suggested earlier, you could include your stretching at the end of a walk or strength-training session.

There are five important stretches:

- hamstring (back of the thigh)
- quadricep (front of the thigh)
- gluteals (bottom)
- shoulder
- chest.

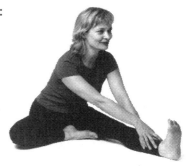

Hamstring (back of the thigh)

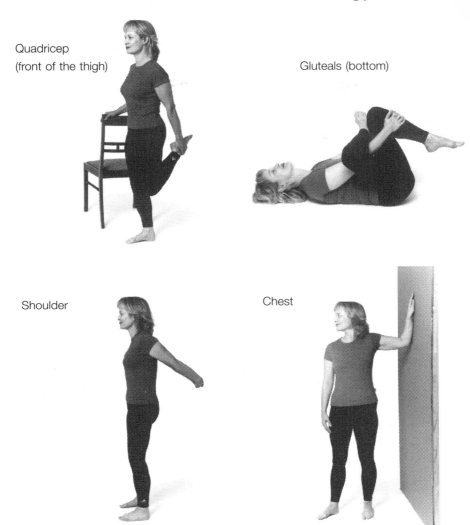

Quadricep
(front of the thigh)

Gluteals (bottom)

Shoulder

Chest

Remember:

- Stretching should be done slowly in a controlled manner.
- Avoid bouncy, ballistic movements.
- Hold each stretch for 15–20 seconds, alternating each side.
- Repeat 3–4 times on each side.
- As you breathe out, relax and move deeper into the stretch.

Stretching doesn't have to be done as part of an exercise session. You may want to do them on the floor while watching television. Your family will get used to it and might even join in. Try stretching on the bedroom floor before you go to bed and enjoy the relaxed feeling afterwards.

Yoga is an excellent way to improve flexibility as well as teaching you some wonderful meditating techniques. Plenty of classes cater for the beginner, so give it a go!

Learning how to relax is important in controlling stress. If you use the time you spend stretching to slow down and relax, it can become a very enjoyable part of your overall exercise program. Relaxation exercises and learning how to breathe deeply can also be very beneficial in controlling hot flushes.

Chapter 11

Pelvic floor exercises

You are probably already aware of the problems associated with a 'weak bladder' and the impact this can have on your life. One in three women suffer from some form of 'leakage' or incontinence and this only increases as they get older. Many women don't seek treatment because they believe it is an inevitable part of having children or they are too embarrassed. Left untreated, however, these symptoms can influence the quality of life now and into the future. Sixty per cent of women in nursing homes are not there because of decreased mental function, but because incontinence severely restricts their lives.

But there is good news. Any form of leakage is not normal and should not be tolerated. With some simple exercises you can stop the situation getting any worse and usually stop the symptoms altogether.

It's important to understand how the waterworks system operates to see how we can improve the problem. Urine is stored in the bladder where it is emptied out through a small tube called the urethra. Urine does not just dribble out; it is pushed out by a bladder muscle called the detrusor muscle. You have no voluntary control over this muscle.

What you do have control over are the pelvic floor muscles and urethral sphincter. The pelvic floor muscles act like a sling supporting the bladder, uterus and bowel. The urethral sphincter is like a drawstring that can tighten to stop urine leaking from the bladder to the urethra, the tube that takes urine through the perineum (the area between your legs). Think of your bladder as a funnel where urine collects and the urethra as the spout. The urethral sphincter tightens around the base of the funnel and the spout, to prevent any liquid escaping.

The pelvic floor muscles not only support these organs (bladder, uterus and bowel) but also help the urethral sphincter to close off the opening of the bladder to the urethra. To stop urine leaking out, the urethral sphincter and pelvic floor muscles contract. To allow urine to pass through they both need to relax. When they relax, the bladder muscle (detrusor muscle) contracts, pushing the urine out.

Don't worry if the anatomy seems confusing—just try to get a general idea how the system functions. If you can understand how it works, you will see how simple it can be to improve the problem.

The main damage is usually done during pregnancy and childbirth. Leakage problems might present themselves after childbirth or not surface until years later. You may have had no problems at all with leakage when, suddenly, at menopause, you start to experience 'accidents'. As you know, menopause is a time when oestrogen levels decrease in the body and this can have a thinning effect on the vagina and urethra. This may cause vaginal dryness, itching and sometimes bleeding. Oestrogen also helps some parts of the bladder and urethra to function properly.

Therefore, menopause is a time to ensure that:

- if you already have problems with leakage (during laughing, coughing or sneezing), going to the toilet frequently or a feeling of urgency, you do not let them get any worse;
- if you don't experience any of these problems, you make sure that problems don't surface in future years.

How do I know I have a problem?

- If you have any sort of leakage it is not normal (no matter what your friends tell you). This includes when coughing, sneezing, jumping or doing physical activity.
- Do you go to the toilet frequently (more than eight times per day)?
- Do you know every 'Ladies' in town, so you won't get caught out?
- Do you find yourself going 'just in case'?

> **Other factors leading to urinary problems**
>
> - Constipation (straining and pushing put pressure on the pelvic floor muscles).
> - Chronic coughing.
> - Overweight (the more you are overweight the more pressure on your pelvic floor muscles).
> - Excess caffeine or alcohol.
> - Ageing (decreased mobility can cause more 'accidents').

- Do you often have a feeling of urgency—where you feel that if you didn't go you would wet your pants?

If you're nodding your head then chances are you are setting in place patterns that will make the problem worse now and in the future. There is no doubt that you can improve the situation, no matter what age you are. A 75-year-old woman can benefit from pelvic floor exercises and bladder retraining. Every woman should include pelvic floor exercises into her daily routine. It is an investment in quality of life.

What can I do about it?

It depends on your situation.

- If you do not experience any problems with leakage, frequency or urgency, then include pelvic floor exercises daily.
- If you are already experiencing leakage, frequency or urgency you will definitely benefit from these exercises. You will also benefit greatly from seeing a qualified physiotherapist or health nurse that specialises in urinary continence (believe me they do exist). They will be able to identify where the problem is coming from and give you an individualised program that will give you the best results.

Pelvic floor exercises strengthen the pelvic floor muscles and urethral sphincter that we discussed above. The pelvic floor muscles are like any other muscle—when they are exercised they respond by getting stronger.

To find out where your pelvic floor muscles are, lie in a propped-up position on a bed or couch. Think of how you would stop the flow of urine if you were emptying your bladder, and try to squeeze the muscles you would use (don't squeeze your buttocks). Hold for three seconds. Relax and rest for ten seconds. Then squeeze and hold for ten seconds (or as long as you can). Relax for ten seconds. Make sure you are not holding your breath—breathe normally. It is important that you do both the fast contractions and the slow ones. The fast squeezes will help when you need a quick, strong force to stop leakage when you cough or sneeze. The slow ones will help with the constant load of keeping urine in the bladder and supporting your abdominal organs. Try to do these exercises twice a day.

Now you know what to do, you need to remember to do them. If you anchor them around certain meal times and do them before and after that meal, it will help to remind you. Another trick is to put red dots around the house or workplace. Whenever you see these dots it's a reminder to do your pelvic floor exercises. Try doing them every time you do the washing up (that's if you don't have a dishwasher).

Like any exercise, you need to ensure that you slowly increase the

---

Pelvic muscle exercise plan

Week 1: five fast contractions and ten long contractions twice each day
Total = 30 contractions each day.
Week 2: five fast contractions and 15 long contractions twice each day
Total = 40 contractions each day.
Week 3 and thereafter: five fast contractions and 20 long contractions twice each day.
Total = 50 contractions each day.
Source: Sampselle et al., 2001

amount and the length of time you do it for, otherwise your body gets used to doing the same thing. As you feel yourself getting stronger, increase the number of fast squeezes that you do. Do the same with the slow squeezes and also increase the length of time that you hold them for.

As well as doing pelvic floor exercises, it is important that you change any learned habits that might be contributing to the problem. These are habits to avoid:

- Going to the toilet 'just in case'.
- Restricting your fluids—make sure you drink 2 litres of water a day.
- Straining when you empty your bowels.

This is a very important issue for all women, particularly during menopause and beyond. It's a problem that can cause loss of self-esteem and confidence and really impact on your quality of life. If you are already experiencing leakage of any kind, seek further help. A trained physiotherapist or health nurse can guide you through each step and ensure that you are doing the exercises correctly. I have outlined a very basic level of exercise but there is so much that can be done to help you. Don't accept urinary problems as a normal part of a woman's life, because it does not have to be that way. Take control of it.

Physiotherapist Pauline Chiarelli specialises in urinary incontinence and has written an easy-to-read book that outlines how you can improve this problem. *Women's Waterworks: Curing Incontinence* is published by the Health Books group and is an excellent follow-up book for you to read.

12

How to get started

The first thing you need to do is make a decision to include exercise in your lifestyle. Without a conscious commitment, exercise will become a fitness fad that is started with enthusiasm but fizzles out when obstacles get in the way. It always concerns us when we hear people say they are starting a 'fitness kick'. Unfortunately, this signals that they will probably not stick to it for long. Including exercise in your lifestyle should be a long-term focus and this is the first commitment you need to make to yourself.

Ask yourself these questions.

1. Do I value the benefits that I will achieve through exercising?
   - Increased cardiovascular fitness.
   - Improved strength, balance and bone density.
   - Slimmer, more toned body shape.
   - Increased energy and sense of well-being.
   - Improved confidence and self-esteem.
2. Am I prepared to set aside time to exercise each week?
   - 30–50 minutes, three to five times a week.
3. What has stopped me from exercising in the past?
   - Not enough time/too busy.
   - I don't like exercise.
   - It's too expensive.
   - I want to lose weight first.

- I've got a bad back/knee/etc.
- I don't have the right clothes. I would look out of place.

There should be no problem answering the first two questions. Believe it or not, you do have time to do three to five sessions a week. The obstacles in question three are the ones you really need to work through, because they are the factors that will crop up again.

Not enough time

We all have 24 hours in our day. How we use them is up to each individual. If exercise is a priority for you then you will allocate time in your day for it. We figure that if the Prime Minister can fit exercise into his schedule we have no excuse. Get up half an hour earlier, use your lunch hour a couple of times a week, set times aside in your diary at the beginning of the week for exercise, arrange to meet someone.

I don't like exercise

This is usually because you have never really exercised consistently before and experienced the real benefits of exercise. If you really hate exercise, give it time. Don't go too hard too fast—start slowly and build gradually. Pick something that you enjoy to start with.

It's too expensive

This is simply not true. You have an exercise option that will cost you absolutely nothing. Start walking (use a comfortable pair of shoes that you already have) and include the strength training exercises that do not use any equipment. All it costs is your time and motivation.

I want to lose weight first

This is a very common feeling among women. They feel that by waiting until they lose weight, they will be able to cope with the exercise better. Losing body fat (which is what you are really trying to achieve) is difficult to do without exercise. You should be thinking of changing your lifestyle by improving your diet and including regular exercise. No matter how much weight you want to lose, exercise should be started from the onset.

I've got a bad back

If you have a problem with your back, you should be exercising to help strengthen the area. This goes for knees, shoulders and neck too. You will definitely benefit from having an exercise professional work out a program for you. This is not an excuse for you to avoid exercising.

I don't have the right clothes

Wear what you feel comfortable in; grab a T-shirt and a pair of shorts. If you are planning on using a fitness centre you will find plenty of women just like you who aren't there for a fashion parade. You might prefer a female-only centre.

If you have other hurdles that tend to get in your way, think about what you can do to surmount them. Sometimes the hardest step is actually identifying what the hurdles are and admitting that these are a problem. Usually the biggest problem is motivation—deciding that you *want* to include exercise in your lifestyle.

> *I can change my life by changing the attitudes of my mind.*
>
> Gus Mercurio

Your sort of exercise

Decide what kind of exercise you want to do. Choose something that you enjoy. If you like swimming, then use swimming as your cardio-vascular exercise. If walking suits you better, grab the dog and head out the door. As outlined earlier, ideally you should combine cardiovascular or aerobic exercise with a strength-training program. The emphasis is on *ideally*. If it seems too much to deal with at first, don't let that put you off. Start anything, as long as you're moving.

Sample program

Cardiovascular/aerobic exercise

Walking is an easy form of exercise to start with and can be done by anyone. Start with 15 minutes three times a week and build up to 45 minutes three to five times a week over a couple of months.

Strengthening exercises

After four to six weeks of walking, look at introducing some strength training into your program. You can follow the exercises outlined in this book or seek the help of an exercise professional. Decide whether you are going to do your strengthening exercises at home or at a fitness centre or studio.

If you decide to exercise at home, will you do it on your own or with a fitness trainer? If you choose to work alone, follow the exercises outlined in this book. If you decide you need help, a fitness trainer can design a program for you.

At a fitness centre, you can work on your own, or an instructor can demonstrate your initial program. Or you might choose to work with a group or a fitness trainer. Working with others builds motivation and encourages you to challenge yourself.

Aim to do strengthening exercises two or three times a week.

A woman's story

At 48 years old, Sandra had little energy and felt sluggish all the time. She was experiencing hot flushes and having difficulty sleeping, and her doctor suggested she take HRT to relieve these symptoms. She decided she would prefer not to take HRT so her doctor recommended some lifestyle modifications, including adjustments to her diet (more soy products) and exercise to help increase her energy levels. Her doctor also recommended she do some weight-bearing exercise to help maintain her bone density.

Personal fitness trainers

We usually associate personal trainers with the rich and famous. You may not realise that many ordinary people are using exercise professionals to help them introduce exercise into their lives or to get the most out of their efforts. The benefits of using a personal fitness trainer are enormous. A trainer will look at your lifestyle and help you make changes that will achieve your goals. This might be through diet and exercise. They will work with you where you choose, at home or in a fitness centre, and will design a program for you that caters for your individual needs. A fitness trainer is there to support, guide and motivate you.

For the price of a facial, you can have an exercise professional come to your house and take you through your exercises, making sure that you are doing them properly. This may be a one-off occasion to get you started, or once a fortnight to keep you on track.

You don't know where to start looking for a trainer? Ring your local fitness centre and ask if they have any trainers they can recommend. Look in the telephone directory: most trainers are listed in the health and fitness section. Ask for an introductory consultation where you can meet the trainer and ask any questions you may have. Most trainers will provide a free introductory session. Don't be afraid to ask their qualifications and for client referrals. Above all, choose a trainer you feel comfortable with.

Sandra had never been much of an exerciser, and the thought of going into a gym with lycra-clad young bodies frightened her. She also knew that it was important for her to start exercising to help keep her bones strong. Sandra had heard a lot about osteoporosis and knew that this was a critical time for losing bone strength.

She decided to start walking three mornings a week before she went to work. At first, it was difficult getting up that little bit earlier and she found it hard to get motivated. Fifteen minutes was all she could handle to start with, but she was surprised how quickly she improved. After a month she could walk for 35 minutes and added a fourth walk at the weekend. She couldn't believe the difference in her energy levels—she'd thought the exercise would make her more tired, but it had the opposite effect. The hot flushes had decreased and her sleeping was better. She no longer felt she was dragging herself through the day.

Sandra had heard that weight training was beneficial for women wanting to maintain strength and bone density and decided to try it for herself. She wanted to find someone to help with her plans. She looked in the phone book and found the names of a couple of fitness trainers. She felt a bit anxious about ringing them as she thought they would only be interested in young people. However, after speaking to a few she organised a time to meet one that she felt comfortable with.

After the initial meeting Sandra felt a lot more relaxed and comfortable about working with a trainer and began seeing her once a week at home. Sandra did the exercises the trainer set her when she came back from her walk—it took her 45 minutes to do both. After a month Sandra decided to see her trainer once a month to keep her on track, and that extended to every two months after a while.

Sandra felt she had a new lease on life. She was fitter and stronger than she had been in her whole life. Everyone told her she looked great—she had lost weight and had toned up her body. Sandra had made positive life changes and began to care more about herself. Her confidence increased as she faced the hurdles of exercise. The fear of approaching a trainer, the cost of sessions and her low fitness were all challenges Sandra faced and overcame. Above all she had control. Sandra was managing her menopause.

Exercise plans

The table below outlines the types of exercises that are going to be most beneficial to you and how often you should be doing them. But how does that translate into your everyday life?

Type of exercise	*Frequency*
Cardiovascular/aerobic	3–5 times/week
Strength training	2–3 times/week
Flexibility	3–5 times/week
Pelvic floor	Daily

Here are three women's exercise plans, showing how they each include exercise in their life.

Plan A

Three mornings a week, Sally gets up an hour earlier to allow her to do her exercise. She goes for a 30-minute walk around her neighbourhood then spends half an hour doing strength exercises and stretching in the courtyard downstairs. At first she was tempted to turn off the alarm, but now she finds she automatically wakes on exercise mornings and is out of bed before the alarm goes off. On Sunday she meets a friend and they go for a longer walk (45–60 minutes). She knows that the arrangement to meet a friend makes sure she doesn't slack off. They have even decided to take part in a 5-km Fun Run/Walk being held in six weeks' time.

Plan B

Cathy started walking about two months ago and, when she felt she was ready, joined a fitness centre so they could help her with some strength exercises. Twice a week Cathy goes to the gym and does a variety of cardiovascular, strength and stretching exercises. She has never used weights before and was a little self conscious about being able to do it. The fitness professional showed her exactly what she was meant to be doing and is monitoring her progress. Cathy goes after work on Wednesday and slips off in her lunch break on Friday. Even after just six weeks of doing the program, she can't believe the improvement in her strength.

Plan C

Pam has been exercising regularly for over 12 months. She started with walking and then included Strength Program 1 (outlined in Chapter 10). After a couple of months she purchased some weights and moved to Program 2. Six months ago she decided to overcome her fear of water and enrolled in an adult learn-to-swim class. This was a big jump for Pam as she has always been terrified of the water. She found there were plenty of other people in the same situation and now Pam is swimming half a kilometre with a goal of 1 km by the end of the year.

Pam has always been a bit of a worrier, and she felt that teaching herself how to relax would help keep her stress levels down. She talked a friend into starting a beginners' yoga class with her and they go once a week. Pam loves the variety of doing different activities and feels better than she has for years.

Checkpoints

- If you have not been exercising for a while it's a good idea to check with your doctor to ensure there are no health conditions that you need to take into account. I'm sure they will be delighted that you are planning to include exercise in your lifestyle.
- Listen to your body and, if you are feeling faint or dizzy, stop. This is different from feeling 'a bit puffed and sweaty'.
- Exercise regularly and build up slowly. Remember: slow and steady wins the race.
- Add variety to your exercise routine. We all get bored if we do the same thing all the time. Even changing the pool you swim at (alternate between 25- and 50-metre pools) can make the exercise session feel totally different.
- Try to exercise with a partner or group at least once a week. It will help you keep on track if you know you have arranged to meet with others.
- Set yourself some goals and write them down. This will give you something to work towards. Maybe a charity walk with a friend,

a bushwalking weekend, or being able to swim 1 km in three months' time.

- If you stop exercising, don't despair. Think about why you stopped, work out what you can do to keep yourself motivated, and start again.
- Above all, maintain a positive attitude to exercise. Do what you enjoy and reap the lifelong benefits to your quality of life.

Summary of Step 3

We have given you a lot of information about exercising during menopause. Let's summarise this to pull it all together. What are the benefits of exercise for me during menopause and beyond?

- Maintains strong bones.
- Strengthens your muscles.
- Maintains your sense of balance.
- Helps you maintain your weight.
- Minimises lifestyle diseases.
- Increases your confidence and self-esteem.

Questions and answers

Q. *I am 52 years old and have never really exercised before. Am I too old to get any benefit from it?*

A. You are never too old to start exercise! No matter what your age you will benefit physically and emotionally from exercise. Your age and current fitness determines what level you start at, but in no way stops you from starting. Walking is a good place to begin. Start slowly and build up gradually.

Q. *I have a bad back and am concerned that I will make it worse if I exercise.*

A. If you have back problems it is even more important that you do regular exercise to help strengthen your muscles and maintain flexibility. Seek professional advice from a physiotherapist or fitness professional about what type of exercise you would benefit from most.

Q. *I have become self-conscious about exercising because I sometimes leak urine if I move suddenly. Also, I don't want to walk too far from home as sometimes I need to go to the toilet suddenly.*

A. What you describe is very common but not often talked about. Don't accept what you are experiencing as something you have to live with. There is a lot that can be done to improve your situation and prevent it from getting worse. Seek out a physiotherapist or nurse who specialises in urinary incontinence to help you overcome this problem. If you leave it untreated it will impact on many areas of your quality of life.

Step 3

Q. *I have read how weight training is very beneficial for maintaining strong bones and muscles—but won't I hurt myself lifting those heavy dumbbells?*

A. People of all ages can do strength training. You start doing the exercises with a light weight and as your muscles get stronger you slowly begin to increase the weight. An 80-year-old woman can start strength training and benefit from it. The key is to build up gradually over time.

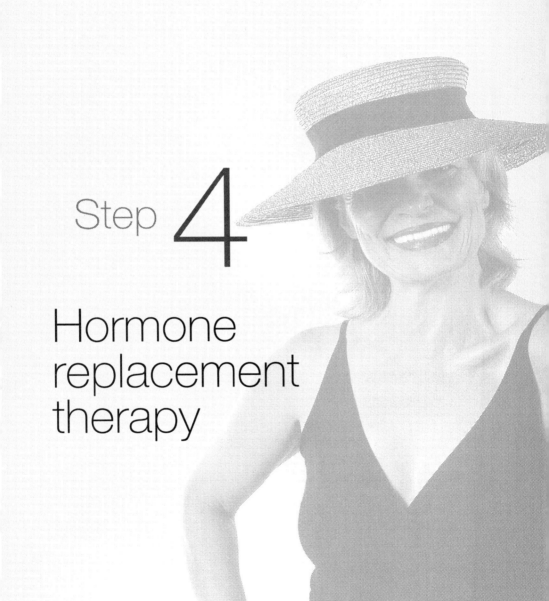

Step 4

Hormone replacement therapy

In Step 4 we take you through the latest research on hormone replacement therapy (HRT). We explore the differences between using it for a short while and for many years; we look at what research is saying about HRT and relief of symptoms; and we discuss HRT and its relationship to bone and heart health, and cancer.

The information on this topic is extensive and confusing. We have tried to simplify it for you to enable you to weigh up the evidence for yourself as an individual, and make the right choice for *you*.

Chapter 13

HRT: to use or not to use?

There is no more controversial topic in women's health today than hormone replacement therapy. The debate about HRT is filled with disagreement and the details are confusing for many women. Here we attempt to simplify the research data to help you understand the evidence for and against HRT.

At every seminar and fitness consultation that we have conducted for women of this age group, we have learned of the absolute confusion about HRT and surrounding issues. It was apparent that, for women from about 45 years of age, one question was of supreme importance: Should I take HRT?

At the end of every menopause seminar that we conduct through Women's Health Qld Wide, women and health professionals line up to ask questions. The same question was asked repeatedly: *Could you just tell me quietly... would you take HRT?* My answer was always the same: *I will not tell you.*

We do not want to influence your decision about taking HRT. We want *you* to make a choice based on *you*—that includes your genetic background, your risk of cardiovascular disease, osteoporosis and breast cancer, and any symptoms that you may experience.

Our goal, therefore, is to give you the latest researched information about HRT and empower you to make the right decision for yourself as an individual. We provide you with research findings from acknowledged sources like the World Health Organization and the International Menopause Society to help you develop a 'feel' for how HRT might best be used.

HRT explained

Many people would like to be able to take one magic tablet that will delay or stop the natural ageing process and make them youthful forever. When HRT was first introduced, many people believed that we had that tablet. HRT was linked with everything that was desireable, from glowing youthful skin to feeling wonderful. It was prescribed in large amounts for women across Europe, the United States and Australia. The fairy tale ended when it was found that it increased the risk of cancer of the uterus. The early type of HRT was ERT (oestrogen alone) and many doctors stopped prescribing it, which consequently decreased dramatically the number of women taking it.

For this reason the HRT prescribed today includes progestogens (the synthetic form of the hormone progesterone), which counteract the effects of oestrogens on the endometrium (the lining of the uterus) and thus decrease the risk of endometrial cancer. HRT (oestrogens plus progestogens) has increased in popularity again and is one of the choices that women can make for use in their menopausal and postmenopausal years.

Hormone replacement therapy (HRT) is the administration of a combination of oestrogens and progestogens together or, sometimes, oestrogens alone.

Our bodies produce chemicals, called hormones, which have very particular effects. The role of the hormone called oestrogen is to keep the female reproductive system in shape, and it also plays a large role in looking after the bones and heart. Oestrogen is produced by the ovaries and around the time of menopause the ovaries start producing less. This can result in long-term changes in heart and bone health (see Chapter 9) and may also produce short-term or temporary changes (menopausal symptoms) while the body is adjusting to the new level of oestrogen.

Progesterone (the other hormone involved in menopause) is also produced by the ovaries. This hormone is important for preparing the lining of the uterus each month in anticipation of pregnancy occurring.

At menopause there is a slow decrease in oestrogen and other hormones in the body. HRT is one of several options for women during and after menopause to increase the levels of oestrogen and progesterone in the body.

HRT usually consists of:

- oestrogen combined with regular levels of progestogen. The progestogen is taken for 10–14 days each month and may result in bleeding similar to a period, less regular bleeding, or none at all; or
- continuous combined oestrogen and progestogen taken every day without any break and with no bleeding; or
- oestrogen alone for women who have had a hysterectomy;
- testosterone for loss of libido, normally combined with any of the above.[1]

How do I get it?

As HRT is a prescription-only medication, you will need to consult a doctor to discuss your options. Your doctor will want to consider your reasons for taking HRT as this can influence the length of time that you will take it.

The decision to use HRT or not should be a shared decision between you and your doctor. Choose a health professional who can provide you with good quality information on the risks and benefits of HRT.

The latest information can take up to two years to reach health professionals. Often research findings are presented at a conference among peers and then submitted for publication in a journal. This process can take one to two years, and then health professionals need to access that information and include the latest findings in their practice. It is also very difficult for health professionals to keep up with the latest findings on everything. General practitioners see a wide range of patients with many different problems, and being up to date with the latest on every specialty is not always possible.

It is for this reason that we encourage you in *The Menopause Made Simple Program* to begin with Step 1, *Health information*. Doctors do not usually mind when patients access the latest information. With the resources available through the Internet today, it is quite appropriate for you to acquire good quality information and share it with your health professional.

Doctors and communication

We have found that the type of communication women experience when they visit a health professional is very important. Research shows that a large number of women do not fill their HRT prescription after they have been given it by the doctor. Exploring the reasons further, many said that they were 'put on HRT', with some women requesting it and others not wanting the prescription at all. A third group, however, had a very positive experience and felt empowered by their choice to take HRT.

Here are two quite different experiences of a consultation about menopause.

My doctor is female and very concerned with women's health, particularly menopause, and has explained the changes taking place in my body to my satisfaction. She took a lot of time to explain and asked me to decide what I wanted to help me make up my mind to take HRT or not. (Monique)

I thought the doctor was impatient, and also that menopause was not particularly important to him. He gave me a prescription for HRT. I had no idea what the side effects were, so I threw it in the bin after leaving his office. (Julie)

Remember, you are under no obligation to return to a health professional where you feel that the service was less than adequate, just as you wouldn't for any other service that you pay for. Women's Health Centres can provide you with names of health professionals that other women have been to and recommend. You are in the driver's seat for your menopause experience, so feel free to seek out a health professional that suits your individual health needs. Your decision to take HRT should occur only after a receptive and informative consultation with your health professional.

What are the ways of taking HRT?

There are several ways of taking HRT:

- tablets, usually taken every day
- skin patches
- gels
- vaginal creams
- vaginal tablets
- vaginal rings.

Choose the way you feel most comfortable with. Many women don't like the idea of taking a tablet every day but feel comfortable rubbing a gel into the skin. The choice is yours.

Several types of oestrogen and progestogen preparations are used in HRT. Some of their components are different and can have varying effects on the way HRT works in your body. Individual women also differ in the way they respond to HRT. Your dosage may differ from that taken by other women and your doctor will advise on the most appropriate strength for you. Remember that it can take some months to adjust to HRT, so if you decide to take it give it a few months to work to get the best effect. A proportion of women cannot tolerate HRT and they will need to explore the other options available to them to relieve their symptoms.

Here are two women's experiences of using HRT:

I had bad symptoms of the hot flushes and headaches and that sort of thing. Since I have been on HRT, I haven't had any of the symptoms that you hear of. (Sue)

HRT obviously worked for Sue, but for Janet it was a different story:

The patches didn't work. I came out in great massive welts and I had to shift the patch every 12 hours from one place to another. Then they put me on the tablets. Anyway, I've been taking it now for three years and I've still got every one of my symptoms! (Janet)

Chapter 14

Short-term use vs long-term use

When you explore the option of taking HRT, you need to consider this question carefully: are you taking HRT for short-term relief of menopausal symptoms (one to two years) and/or are you taking HRT for perceived long-term health benefits (five years and over)?

Whether to use HRT for a short or long term is a disputed question. Researchers and health professionals have battled with this question for many years, with conflicting opinions. For this reason a Clinical Synthesis Conference, held in Milan, Italy, was organised in June 1999, by major medical and academic bodies. The aim of the meeting was to bring together research from around the world to come up with recommendations for the best use of HRT. Their conclusions for the short- and long-term use of HRT included the following:

Short–term use

> *Use of HRT for a few years at around the time of the menopause will relieve menopausal symptoms and not lead to a substantial increase or decrease in cancer, cardiovascular disease, or osteoporosis.*

Long–term use

> *Although there is considerable evidence about the health effects of long-term use of HRT, on average the balance between the risk and benefits*

is not overwhelming in either direction. For many women the benefits of long-term HRT will outweigh the risks; for others risks outweigh the benefits. The use of HRT has to be tailored to the needs and desires of the individual.[2]

Short-term use of HRT

What are the short-term benefits of HRT?

The main aim of HRT is to relieve menopausal symptoms and it is highly effective for women with typical menopausal symptoms. The reasons that doctors should prescribe HRT in the short term is for hot flushes and night sweats and changes to the vagina and genitalia region which may result in a feeling of vaginal dryness.

In the short term, both oestrogen replacement therapy and HRT will improve hot flushes, vaginal dryness and some sleep disturbances. HRT is also useful in early menopause.

Hot flushes

Research has shown that all types of HRT will reduce hot flushes. The method of taking it isn't important.

Vaginal dryness and urethral irritability

Urogenital symptoms (e.g. dry vagina, maybe some urinary difficulties) are improved by taking HRT orally or vaginally. Improvements in this area are seen within weeks, but it is important to remember that it will take months of treatment to achieve the full benefit.

Sleep disturbances

HRT is effective in relieving sleep disturbances that are due to hormonal changes in your body. (It will not help if your reason for poor sleep is the noisy neighbours, worry about paying the bills or the uncomfortable mattress you sleep on.)

Early menopause

A small group of women will have an early menopause (25–40 years). Early menopause occurs as a result of surgery or treatment that affects the ovaries. Please note: having a hysterectomy will not bring on an early menopause unless the ovaries are also removed. A hysterectomy involves removing the uterus (a sac-like organ that does not produce any hormones, and so it has nothing to do with your menopause).

Early menopause usually produces severe symptoms and special attention should be given to the use of HRT. With early menopause you will need to consult a specialist who will give you the best advice on your HRT options. Women who have an early menopause are well advised to consider taking HRT, at least until the time that their natural menopause would have started.

Side effects of short-term use

- *Breast tenderness.* A small group of women who take HRT develop breast tenderness. Some women get it quite severely, others only slightly. Many women describe this tenderness as the same as premenstrual tenderness of the breasts. No doubt, the oestrogen in the HRT affects the breast tissue, making it more dense than before. This tenderness often subsides after a few months and it may be worth persevering if you want to take HRT.
- *Breakthrough bleeding (spotting).* This annoying side effect can be controlled. Discuss it with your doctor who can adjust the type, level and way of administering the HRT. Remember, it can take a few months to sort out the best regime of HRT for your use.
- *Venous thromboembolism.* Venous thromboembolism occurs when a thrombus (a mass of a substance called fibrin) forms in the deep veins of the legs (deep vein thrombosis, DVT).

  It is a major potential complication of short-term (1–2 years) HRT use. The risk of developing an embolism increases very slightly in the first few years of HRT use.

  In your consultation with your health professional about taking HRT, it is important that your personal and family history of deep vein thrombosis is discussed. Also, your weight should be measured. Obesity has been shown to be a risk factor for developing a DVT.

There may be no signs at all of a DVT—it may just sit there and cause no symptoms. Occasionally, it may cause chest pain or breathlessness, and you may feel a throbbing at the back of your leg. Make a point of knowing the signs.

Surgery can increase the risk of developing a DVT so, if you are to have surgery, discuss with the surgeon the fact that you are taking HRT.

If you are taking a 'long haul flight' (i.e. flying halfway round the world), you are advised to take low-dose aspirin to help decrease any slight risk of DVT.[3]

* *Weight gain.* Women express major concern about weight gain when taking HRT.

> *I believed that HRT would cause my breasts to become swollen and painful and that I would also put on weight. (Linda)*

The research concludes that HRT *does not* cause weight gain. Women in this age group tend to change their exercise and eating habits and it is these changes that are associated with the weight gain. Steps 2 and 3 of this book show you how to reverse those eating and exercise habits so that you can throw out that weight problem.

HRT and psychological health

As we discussed in Step 1, symptoms such as depression, nervous tension, palpitations, lack of energy, fluid retention, difficulty in concentrating and dizzy spells appear to be related to ageing and occur commonly in men as well as women.

Despite these findings, medical and public pressure for the use of HRT in the treatment of psychological symptoms of menopause still exists, with some medical experts supporting its use. Some clinicians continue to promote the notion that a woman gets depressed during menopause, and prescribe and encourage the use of HRT for its treatment. The manufacturers of HRT preparations, in an advertising campaign in Canada in 1990, listed anxiety and irritability among the list of menopausal symptoms for which HRT could be used.

However, research literature concludes that depression and anxiety do not respond well to hormone replacement therapy, and for some women:

> ... the greatest benefit of a menopause clinic may come not from any specific hormonal or drug treatment but from the interest and support of the staff.[4]

HRT for the long term

To understand the issues of long-term use of HRT, it is important that we take a step back in history to explore why there is still controversy in some areas.

Most of the evidence that we have about HRT use comes from studies that are conducted on a group of women at one point in time (cross-sectional studies). In a cross-sectional study, a group of women is studied over a short period of time. These studies are very important and can provide excellent information on an issue, but they cannot tell us what would happen over a long period of time.

A cross-sectional study may be conducted, for example, to test how HRT affects cholesterol levels. It may find that HRT acts in a positive way, but that doesn't tell us how it would act if it was taken for ten years. We can assume that because it works well over a short period of time, it may work well over ten years, but we don't really know until we have studied the same women over the longer time period. Long-term studies (longitudinal studies) may often reveal something that might not have been accounted for in a short-term study. The information they provide is often very valuable.

Currently, several large long-term trials are being carried out to explore the role of hormones in the development of breast cancer, osteoporosis and cardiovascular disease. The main studies are:

- The Women's Health Initiative
- The Postmenopausal Estrogen/Progestin Intervention (PEPI) Trial
- The Heart and Estrogen–Progestin Replacement Study (HERS)
- The Women's International Study of Long Duration Oestrogen after Menopause (WISDOM)
- The Million Women Study.

Only the PEPI trial and the HERS study have been completed. So as you can see we actually have quite a way to go before we can speak conclusively about the long-term risks and benefits of HRT use by women. It's suggested that we will not have the definitive answers to long-term HRT use until around 2010.

However, in the appendix at the end of the book, we have given you the web addresses of these large studies, which constantly update the findings from the large trials. Often they will analyse the results for the first three years, say, and release this information to give women and health professionals an idea of what is happening. With this information you will have the latest facts on what research is saying about HRT. It is important that you are knowledgeable about the health information in this area, as it is still a long way from being conclusive.

Chapter 15

HRT: risks and benefits

Cancer is common in women from developed countries, with breast cancer being the most common cancer. More than 80 per cent of cancers diagnosed in women occur after the age of 50 years. Cancer is the most common cause of death in women aged between 50 and 60 years. After 60 years cardiovascular disease becomes the most common cause of death. You can see that this decade of a woman's life (50–60 years) is a time when women need to be vigilant about screening and prevention programs for breast, endometrial and cervical cancers.

HRT and breast cancer

According to the World Health Organization, one of the most controversial aspects of HRT is its possible association with an increased risk of breast cancer.

Breast cancer is the most common malignant disease in women from developed countries (excluding Japan), with the incidence increasing all over the world, including areas of previously low incidence such as Asia.

An abundance of studies has explored the link between HRT and breast cancer since the mid-1970s, although those conducted since 1985 tend to be the most valuable. This is due to the studies including larger number of women and being conducted for longer time periods.

On current evidence, the use of oestrogen and progestogen (HRT) by postmenopausal women may be associated with an increased risk of breast cancer. The increased risk appears to be for women who are currently using HRT or who have recently used it for five years or longer. It appears that this increase rises with longer duration of use. There does not appear to be any significant increase in risk if HRT is used for only a few years (say one to three years).[5]

The risk decreases after HRT is stopped, and past users or women who used it more than five years earlier showed no increased risks.

The breast cancers developed by women taking HRT tend to be localised to the breast (i.e. early-stage cancer) and less advanced than those in women not taking HRT. We don't know why. It may be the type of women who are using HRT, it may be the action of HRT on the cancer or it may be that women who use HRT return often to their doctor to renew scripts and are reminded to have a breast examination, so the cancer is picked up early.

The association of HRT and breast cancer remains an important area of research. Data from large longitudinal studies like The Women's Health Initiative and The Million Women Study are required before definitive answers can be given.

HRT and endometrial cancer

Endometrial cancer (cancer of the lining of the uterus) has the honour of being the first type of cancer to be linked to HRT. This cancer was linked to the oestrogen-only therapy that was prescribed in the early 1970s. More than 30 well regarded studies found large increases in endometrial cancer with the use of oestrogen therapy (ERT). The longer women used it (five years or more) the higher the risk of developing endometrial cancer

The form in which oestrogen-only therapy is taken makes no difference. The World Health Organization states that any use of oestrogen only, by any mode of administration—vaginal, through the skin or intramuscularly—is likely to have similar effects.

Adding progestogen to the oestrogen (HRT) reduces the effect of this increased risk. Postmenopausal women with an intact uterus should use a combination of oestrogen and progestogen to minimise the risk of endometrial cancer.

Research shows that, as with breast cancer, there is little or no risk for the first five years, with the risk increasing slightly with the use for five years or more.[6]

Because women have been using the combined form of HRT (oestrogen and progestogens) for a shorter time, there are fewer data available than for the use of oestrogen alone. It is important, therefore, that the findings discussed above are looked at in the larger studies being conducted, before firm conclusions can be reached.

HRT and cervical cancer

Although it is unlikely that HRT increases the risk of developing cervical cancer, existing data on HRT and cervical cancer are inadequate for evaluation. Very few studies have been conducted in this area that involve large numbers of women. The few that have been performed found no association between HRT and cervical cancers.[7]

HRT and ovarian cancer

The American Cancer Society said in 2001 that the use of HRT slightly increases the risk of developing fatal ovarian cancers after ten years of use. No increase in risk is seen if you use HRT for less than ten years. This risk is low and needs to be considered in the context of the overall risks and benefits in your use of HRT.

HRT and colorectal cancer

Colorectal cancer is a common form of cancer for women in developed countries. Initial studies indicate that using HRT may decrease your risk of developing colorectal cancer. Researchers are not sure, however, whether these results are due to other factors like diet. It is too early to say anything conclusive.

HRT use by women who have had breast or endometrial cancer

There is currently insufficient research data to say whether HRT should be used by women who have had breast or endometrial cancer. Some specialists suggest that it is safe to offer HRT to women who have had breast cancer, while others are totally against it, fearing that it may cause a recurrance. The decision must be made by the woman and her specialist, and HRT should be prescribed only after the woman is made aware of the uncertainty of the risk at present.

HRT use in women who have had endometrial cancer has revealed few problems, and it is suggested that the potential benefits outweigh the risks. More research on the use of HRT in women who have had either breast cancer or endometrial cancer needs to be conducted before any definite recommendations can be made.

HRT and bone health

The main aim in relation to osteoporosis is to prevent it from occurring, and many short-term studies have shown that HRT can prevent bone loss. Studies of the effects of HRT on bone density show that the administration of oestrogen (ERT), or oestrogen plus progestogen (HRT) is effective in maintaining bone density in postmenopausal women.[8]

We don't know whether using HRT will prevent fractures for the rest of a woman's life. What is known, however, is that once HRT is stopped the bone loss returns to the same level as that for women who do not take HRT.

HRT has been shown to be most effective for increasing bone mass in the following circumstances:

- in women over 60 years of age. It appears that the best time to take HRT may not be straight after menopause (i.e. in your fifties), but after 60 years of age. This raises an interesting question about when to start HRT if the only reason you are taking it is to decrease your risk of osteoporosis;
- women who have low bone density;
- cancellous bone (such as the vertebrae in your back) more than cortical bone (such as the femur or leg bones);
- when taken with increased calcium and adequate vitamin D. HRT has been shown to be more effective if it is used with a calcium intake of 1000 mg and vitamin D (for those who are unable to obtain vitamin D naturally from sunlight).

What about HRT use in older age to prevent osteoporosis?

The average age for experiencing a hip fracture is 80 years, so a few years of HRT at menopause will not reduce a woman's chance of

HRT and osteoporosis

- HRT is effective for the prevention and treatment of osteoporosis after menopause for the time that you take it.
- HRT increases bone mineral density (BMD), decreases bone turnover and reduces the risk of fractures. These effects decline rapidly as soon as you stop the treatment. To decrease the risk of hip fracture, HRT will need to be taken in your sixties and probably into your seventies.
- Women who are at high risk of fracture will benefit most from HRT and can easily be identified by their doctor through a bone density measurement.

Source: Clinical Synthesis Conference, 1999

fracturing a hip in later life. If you are taking HRT to prevent osteo-porosis in later life, you need to commit to taking it for a long time—that is, for 20 years or more (after age 60)—to gain the benefits when you need them most (around age 80). Alternatively, if you are taking HRT only to prevent osteoporosis, you may consider starting it at around the age of 65 years.

It makes no difference whether you take HRT in tablet form, in the gel or in a patch. All routes of administration of oestrogens appear to have the same effect on bone density.

HRT and cardiovascular disease

Lots of studies have been undertaken to measure the effect of taking HRT on your heart health. Two long-term studies, HERS and PEPI (see Appendix) have been completed and have released results that have changed the way that doctors look at prescribing HRT to prevent CVD in women.

Heart and Estrogen–Progestin Replacement Study (HERS)

HERS was a US$40 million trial published in 1998 that studied 2760 American women with previous heart disease, such as a myocardial infarction, or with over 50 per cent narrowing of a coronary artery. The study was conducted for a period of about four years, during which time about 170 (12 per cent) women in each group either died from heart disease or suffered a myocardial infarction that was not fatal.[9]

The study concluded that there was an increased risk of a heart attack in the first year of starting HRT, and an increased risk of venous thrombosis and embolism in women taking HRT who had had a previous cardiovascular event (such as a heart attack). Although the results showed a favourable effect on lipids (fats circulating in blood), there was little or no reduction seen in coronary events or deaths. This research didn't look at women who had never had a previous CVD event, so the findings relate only to women who have had, say, a heart attack or stroke prior to starting HRT.[10]

These findings from HERS conflict with results from earlier cross-sectional studies and remind us, as researchers, how important the long-term trials are. Research from these earlier cross-sectional studies suggested that HRT may protect women from CVD so, for a while, doctors prescribed HRT as a drug that would prevent women from developing CVD. Now we realise, however, that there are not enough data from the longitudinal studies (large, long-term studies) to say for certain that HRT should be used for the prevention of CVD. As with other areas of interest, we will need to wait for the results from other long-term studies, due around 2010 and beyond.

In 2000, the International Menopause Society estimated that up to 90 per cent of heart disease could be significantly delayed by adopting lifestyle measures that include a healthy diet and exercise, and ceasing to smoke.[11]

The International Menopause Society includes many of the world's leaders in the field of menopause. It conducted an Expert Workshop in October 2000 to discuss and evaluate the latest research on cardiovascular disease and hormone replacement therapy because of the many controversies that now exist. The Expert Group released a statement to the press in 2000 which said that, after careful consideration of all the research:

> ... there is no clear reason to commence HRT solely or primarily to confer a cardiovascular benefit. Equally there is not compelling evidence for discontinuing or indeed not initiating therapy because of concern of cardiovascular risk. In any case, all medical intervention should be individualised to specific women's characteristics and needs.

HRT and your brain

Studies looking at a possible beneficial effect of HRT on dementia are in the very early stages. They are researching the effect of HRT on the cells of animals, and some suggest that HRT may play a protective role in cognitive decline and dementia. However, the data from the research are insufficient to form any conclusions as yet. This research is ongoing and I am sure we will hear more in future years. In the meantime, there seems no substantial reason for taking HRT to prevent dementia or improve your brain's functioning.

In the short term, it appears that using HRT for up to five years to relieve the symptoms of menopause is a safe and effective option. We also identified a number of large, long-term studies which are exploring the areas of HRT and cancer, osteoporosis, heart and brain health. In some areas, there is enough evidence to say a definite yes or no, while in other areas we will have to wait about ten years for any definite answers.

That is why so much controversy exists around the topic of HRT, because we don't have all the answers yet. What you are able to do now, however, is to read research findings as they are published. Visit the websites of the big studies and have a look at the latest releases.

On the following pages are two flow charts to help you make the choice that is best for you when choosing HRT. One looks at short-term use and the other at long-term use. Remember: no one can really make the choice for you—look at your individual situation and decide what suits you.

Choosing HRT for short-term use

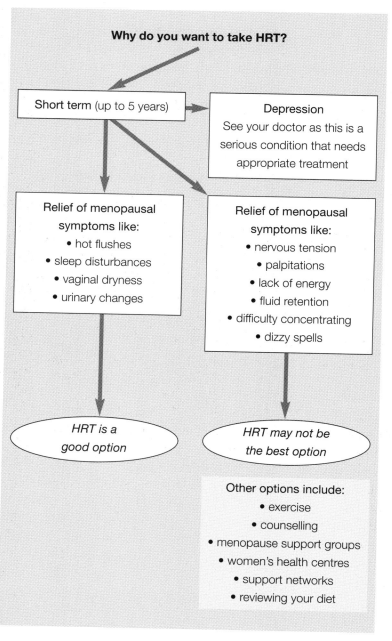

Why do you want to take HRT?

Short term (up to 5 years)

Depression
See your doctor as this is a
serious condition that needs
appropriate treatment

Relief of menopausal
symptoms like:
- hot flushes
- sleep disturbances
- vaginal dryness
- urinary changes

Relief of menopausal
symptoms like:
- nervous tension
- palpitations
- lack of energy
- fluid retention
- difficulty concentrating
- dizzy spells

*HRT is a
good option*

*HRT may not be
the best option*

Other options include:
- exercise
- counselling
- menopause support groups
- women's health centres
- support networks
- reviewing your diet

Step 4

Choosing HRT for long-term use

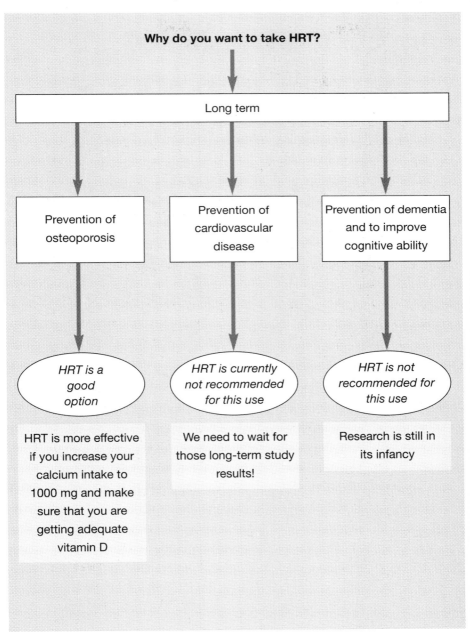

Why do you want to take HRT?

Long term

| Prevention of osteoporosis | Prevention of cardiovascular disease | Prevention of dementia and to improve cognitive ability |

HRT is a good option

HRT is currently not recommended for this use

HRT is not recommended for this use

HRT is more effective if you increase your calcium intake to 1000 mg and make sure that you are getting adequate vitamin D

We need to wait for those long-term study results!

Research is still in its infancy

Step 4

Questions and answers

Q. *I would like to take HRT for about 12 months to relieve hot flushes and vaginal dryness. Will this increase my risk of developing breast cancer?*

A. This is unlikely. Research to date suggests that taking HRT for up to five years results in no significant increase in breast cancer. For the symptoms of hot flushes and vaginal dryness, HRT may be a good option for you.

Q. *I have been prescribed HRT (oestrogen and progestogen) but I don't like taking the progestogen for 12 days each month. Does it matter if I take the oestrogen only?*

A. It is vitally important that you take the progestogen with the oestrogen. Taking oestrogen alone will raise your risk of developing endometrial cancer, unless you have had a hysterectomy and your uterus has been removed.

Q. *Since taking HRT I have gained 6 kg in weight. Is this due to the HRT?*

A. No. Many research trials have shown that HRT does not cause weight gain. What may be happening is that you are holding extra fluid in your body. And there are many other reasons why you may put on weight at this time of your life. Re-read Steps 2 and 3, on eating and exercising, and incorporate the suggestions into your lifestyle—you will soon see that weight disappear.

Step 4

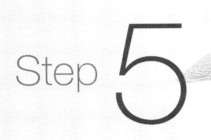

Step 5

Alternatives
to HRT

So you have decided not to take HRT, or you have tried it and it didn't work for you. You are not alone. Recent research found that about 50 per cent of women decided not to take HRT, while a further 25 per cent tried it but, finding that it didn't work for them, stopped taking it. So, about 75 per cent of all women in Western countries choose for one reason or another not to take HRT.

Until recently, women were offered HRT or nothing for menopause. Now women are demanding alternatives and there is evidence that some complementary therapies can be very helpful for menopause. The group of women who choose not to take HRT need their decision to be respected and alternatives offered by health professionals.

In this section we look at all the material that is emerging on complementary therapies for menopause, and provide you with the latest information on their usefulness. Our discussion covers phytoestrogens, natural progestogens and herbal compounds.

Chapter 16

Complementary therapies

Natural therapies take longer to work probably, but if they are effective they're probably a whole lot better for your body because they don't change your metabolism and do funny things to you.

Karen

In the past the term 'alternative medicine' was given to any non-prescribed medicine used by consumers. The words imply working in isolation from mainstream medicine, so that anything that is taken alternatively cannot be taken or practised alongside traditional medicine. A more current term, and one that we think is more appropriate, is 'complementary medicine' which implies that this type of health care can complement traditional health care rather than working in isolation from it.

There is a lot of evidence to suggest that many complementary therapies and medicines can be beneficial for women during menopause. Sometimes, it is not about the choice of, say, taking HRT or an alternative, but looking at all the options and using the right combinations of complementary or traditional medicine for you as an individual.

The use of complementary medicine has grown rapidly in Western countries in the past few years, and it has always been the dominant medicine in many Asian countries. A recent study in Australia showed that almost half the respondents to a survey on the use of complementary medicine had used at least one non-medically prescribed complementary medicine (excluding calcium, iron and prescribed vitamins) in the past year. The survey, conducted in South Australia, also found that about one-fifth of the respondents had visited at least one complementary health practitioner in the past year.[1]

Why is complementary medicine so popular?

First, it seems that a number of people are dissatisfied with the results of traditional medical treatment. They are not happy with the outcome of their prescribed medicine. In the area of menopause, there is a large group of women who try HRT and then stop using it. For various reasons, they are not satisfied with the outcome of taking the traditional medicine, HRT, prescribed by a doctor, and so they seek out alternatives.

A second reason for the increasing use of complementary medicine is that many people are not satisfied with their relationship with their doctor. Women may feel that the doctor does not allow enough time for the consultation, does not listen properly to their concerns and does not provide adequate information about the treatment options available for menopause. Many women have told us of their dissatisfaction with their consultation.

I have actually been told that I'm just getting old and that I should overlook these things. They ... diminish you or trivialise what you're saying to them and they offer you no information whatsoever. She just said go on HRT. (Jody)

The doctors don't tell you anything. They don't say, go to your library and read this book. They just say, this is what you've got to do next. Well, maybe that's not what you want to do next? They don't give you any alternatives—that's what I've found with the medical profession. It seems like they've catalogued everybody, you know. They don't even say, do you know anything about it? They just say, this is the next step. (Trudy)

One of the major pitfalls of complementary medicine is the belief by many women that anything that is natural must be 100 per cent safe.

As with many beliefs, this is not true and it is important that we take the same amount of caution with natural medicines as with prescribed medicines. Most natural medicines and herbs are really prescribed medicines in their rawest form. Most traditional medicines are just refined and manufactured 'natural medicines', which have had to undergo rigorous testing and research before they can be prescribed.

You need to keep this in mind as you sort through the huge amount of material now available on alternatives to HRT and complementary medicines for menopause. Just like HRT, complementary therapies for menopause is turning into big business and you need to act like a detective when searching all the information available so that you can make the decision that is right for you.

Common problems with complementary medicines

There are two common practices when taking complementary medicines. The first is to think that 'more is better'. Women often end up taking more than the recommended dose, believing that, because it is natural, more will not hurt them. This is a dangerous practice as many complementary medicines contain powerful substances which can make you ill if taken in larger doses.

The second common practice with complementary therapies is to 'take them secretly'. Many women choose not to tell their doctor that they are taking additional medicines as they think the doctor might not approve. This is also a dangerous practice as many prescribed drugs can have quite adverse effects if taken with some complementary medicines.

On the other hand, if we think of these medicines as complementary rather than alternative, we may find that a combination of traditional and complementary medicines may work best. Remember, many health professionals use complementary therapies as well as traditional medicines and can work with you to help you achieve an excellent state of health.

Tips for using complementary therapies

- If you have a serious health problem that you have never been to a doctor for, consider having a consultation first to rule out any major health problems.
- Consult a qualified complementary health practitioner to obtain an individual assessment and health care program.
- Choose a complementary health practitioner who is a member of a professional association with a code of ethics, a disciplinary procedure for practitioners who break this code and a complaints procedure for dissatisfied clients. This information can be obtained from the various professional organisations.
- Choose a practitioner with an adequate level of training (at present, except in Victoria where legislation has been introduced requiring Chinese medicine practitioners to be registered, there are no minimum qualifications required to enable people to call themselves naturopaths, herbalists or homoeopaths—only osteopaths and chiropractors have to be officially registered).
- Choose a complementary practitioner who is willing to work with your medical practitioner (if required).
- Know the outcomes they expect from the treatment and ask the practitioner to estimate what length of treatment time is necessary before these outcomes are realised.
- Be wary about practitioners who make guarantees about curing longstanding health problems or who suggest treatments that seem extreme or overly expensive.

Source: Braun, 1999

If you choose to take complementary therapies, treat them the same as you would prescribed drugs—take the recommended dose and let your doctor know what you are taking.

We have looked at the use of complementary medicines in general. The next chapter considers specific treatments for menopause.

Meanwhile, here are some useful websites that you may like to explore on complementary and alternative medicines:

- NIH Office of Dietary Supplements: http://dietary-supplements.info.nih.gov
- National Women's Health Information Centre: www.4woman.gov
- NIH National Centre for Complementary and Alternative Medicine: http://nccam.nih.gov

Chapter 17

Supplements

We mentioned earlier that only about one-quarter of menopausal women use HRT, while the other three quarters do not. What is this large group of women who are not using HRT doing to ease the symptoms of menopause?

Studies have shown that women are using a variety of strategies to combat menopausal symptoms and prevent such problems as osteoporosis and cardiovascular disease. The three things that women said were most useful for them during menopause were:

- exercise
- diet modification
- stress reduction.[2]

Phytoestrogens

In the area of diet, the most frequent suggestions from women included following a healthy diet, taking tofu and/or soy milk and increasing their calcium intake. Exploring further the advice to take tofu and soy milk, we find that these two dietary substances contain high amounts of phytoestrogens.

The use of phytoestrogens by menopausal women is growing rapidly, either by increasing them in the diet or by using phytoestrogen-based supplements. We discussed phytoestrogens in your diet in Step 2, *Eating for menopause*. Supplements are a separate issue because most of the evidence for the benefits of phytoestrogens has come from studying the diets of other cultures. The use of supplements, in the forms of tablets or powder, is a new area that is currently being researched.

Phytoestrogens are naturally occurring compounds found in many foods; they produce similar effects to the oestrogen in the body. Over the last century the Western diet has changed from one that was heavily based on grain and legumes to one that is high in animal protein and unrefined grains. This dietary change means that many Western diets no longer include unrefined fruit, vegetables and grain, where the most phytoestrogens are found. We have inadvertently altered our diet very significantly for the first time in history, and this may be increasing our susceptibility to diseases like breast cancer and cardiovascular problems.

Menopausal symptoms enter the picture when we consider that phytoestrogens are like weak oestrogens, and they would have been consumed in fairly large amounts in the diet in earlier times. Around menopause our level of oestrogen decreases and what may be happening is that women who eat or drink large amounts of phytoestrogens may be helping to increase those levels of oestrogen in the body again.

For this reason, researchers suggest that increasing phytoestrogens, either in your diet or through supplements, may help to decrease menopausal symptoms.

Use around the world

In countries like Japan and China where the people consume large amounts of phytoestrogens, women tend to have fewer menopausal symptoms, as well as less breast cancer and cardiovascular disease, than women from Western countries. Studies that look at populations around the world have found that those who consume large amounts of phytoestrogens in their diet have a lower risk of many of the so-called 'Western diseases'.[3] This is true for both men and women—Asian men are far less likely to get prostate cancer than men from Western countries.

Average isoflavone intake (mg per day)							
Japan	China	India	USA	Spain	UK	Sweden	Finland
38.2	10.6	1.2	0.012	0.01	0.0055	0.0002	0.0001

Source: Husband, 2001

Sources of phytoestrogens

Phytoestrogens are found in a wide variety of plants including cereals, legumes and grasses. Linseed, soy beans and soy products are the richest sources of phytoestrogens. Phytoestrogenes fall into three groups: (1) flavones and isoflavones, (2) the lignans, and (3) coumestans. Phytoestrogen supplements usually contain isoflavones.

It is important to distinguish between the effects of *dietary* phyto-estrogens and those in tablet form. Most of the evidence that says that phytoestrogens are good for us comes from studying people who take them in their diet. When we look at refining phytoestrogens and putting them into a supplement, however, we find that only few studies have been conducted yet on how the supplements work.

Several phytoestrogen supplements are now on the market. The aim of these products is to supply the equivalent of 40 mg of isoflavonoids in a tablet that you take once daily to increase the level of phytoestro-gens in your body. Some research is currently being conducted on how effective these supplements are, and early data show some promising results.

Promensil

Red clover is a valuable source of isoflavones. Promensil is a tablet containing 40 mg of isoflavonoids derived from red clover. Early research has reported an overall reduction in hot flushing after four weeks of use in women taking one tablet per day. There may be other benefits, in the areas of cardiovascular protection and bone loss, but there is no evidence yet.

Caution needed

You need to remember that much of the evidence for believing that phytoestrogens are good for us comes from what is termed 'epidemiological data'. Epidemiological data are gathered when we look at population groups and observe what is happening to them, rather than running a research trial and looking at the differences between two groups. That is why the evidence is stronger for increasing phytoestrogens in your dietary intake rather than through a supplement or tablet.

Asian cultures have been consuming the food they do for a very long time, but phytoestrogens in supplement form is quite a new phenomenon and so the research that is testing the effects of these supplements is also relatively new.

> ### Use of phytoestrogens
>
> - The evidence on the effects of phtyoestrogens is based largely on epidemiological studies (studies looking at groups of people), with very few studies conducted on humans in controlled situations.
> - It may be useful to menopausal and postmenopausal women to consume 45 mg of dietary phytoestrogens daily.
> - Animal studies of dietary phytoestrogens show that many body processes are affected, and the emerging evidence for menopausal women shows that phytoestrogens are beneficial.

Natural progesterone

Natural progesterone products are not actually derived from 'nature' but artificially produced in a laboratory. The term 'natural progesterone' leads many people to believe that the product comes from totally natural ingredients, and so can sometimes be misleading. The term is used to distinguish the product from the synthetic progesterone (progestogen) used in HRT.

Natural progesterone is available in Australia on a doctor's prescription, and some health practitioners recommend it as the supplement of choice instead of using HRT. Because natural progesterone copies the body's progesterone it is important that the dosage is professionally prescribed. That is why it was removed from general sale in Australia and became available by prescription only.

Natural progesterone is available in:

- creams
- vaginal pessaries
- vaginal suppositories
- tablets and capsules.

The recommendation is to use it as a cream or vaginal pessary or suppository. Natural progesterone loses its effectiveness when taken by mouth as it is broken down by the liver.

The cream is applied to areas of the body where the skin is thin, like around the breast and the chest area, as this increases the absorption through the skin. It can take up to three months to have any effect so if you decide to use this option it is best to give it a few months' trial.

What does it do?

This is where the controversy comes in. Tremendous claims have been made about the effectiveness of natural progesterone; it is said to decrease menopausal symptoms, migraine, loss of sex drive and depression. But the research that has been conducted on natural progesterone is scanty and there is not enough evidence yet to support these claims.

Nevertheless, many women use this option and find that it works for them. We don't know exactly what happens with natural progesterone so, if you choose this option, you need to remember to take the same care as you would with any other replacement drug for menopause. Even though it's called 'natural', it is a laboratory-made replacement that needs to be taken accordingly.

Wild yam creams

A lot of confusion surrounds wild yam and natural progesterone. Wild yam does not contain natural progesterone and therefore the cream can be bought over the counter. It contains a type of phytoestrogen that is found in wild yams and soy beans. The effects that some women receive from using wild yam are probably due to an increased level of phyto-estrogens. Wild yam will not increase your progesterone levels.

Women have said that using wild yam creams relieved their menopausal symptoms. A lot of the evidence for using wild yam comes from stories from the women themselves and, while these are impor-tant, further controlled research needs to be conducted before any conclusions can be drawn.

Herbal compounds

I saw a naturopath, and I'm on a herbal mixture for hormones... I've been on it for a month now and I'm feeling so great. I still get a few sweats, but I feel great! (Chris)

Several other plants or herbs are thought to act on the body in the same way as phytoestrogens and therefore have oestrogenic effects. They include dong quai, black cohosh and ginseng, which we look at now. Herbalists or Chinese medical practitioners are best to prescribe these for you as they have experience in working with herbs for the best effect. Be aware, however, that the herbal industry is almost entirely unregu-lated and you need to be prudent when choosing a practitioner.

Dong quai

Dong quai has been used in Chinese medicine for a long time, and is said to be a good herb for premenstrual and menopausal complaints. No conclusive research has been conducted on dong quai, but it is frequently prescribed by herbalists and Chinese medical practitioners. A form of phytoestrogens called coumarins are found in dong quai, which may account for its claimed effects on menopausal symptoms.

Small trials on dong quai were conducted in 1998 by the Natural Therapies Unit at the Sydney Menopause Centre but no significant effects on menopausal symptoms were found.

Dong quai has been made into a supplement called 'Rejuvex' by SunSource, in the form of capsules containing 200 mg of dong quai. This is a new product and very little research has been conducted on it to date.

Black cohosh

Black cohosh is also known as black snakeroot or bugbane. It is thought to contain phytoestrogens and therefore may have similar effects. Black cohosh comes from the medicine of Indigenous Americans where it has been used for many ailments, including menstrual complaints and menopausal symptoms.

Some side effects associated with black cohosh include nausea, vomiting and uterine contractions.

Black cohosh has been turned into a supplement called 'Remifemin', which is claimed to have oestrogenic effects. There have been few scientific studies carried out on this supplement as it is fairly new.

Ginseng

Ginseng is used by herbalists to increase energy and endurance. It is also thought to boost the immune system so that the body can handle the stresses and strains of life more effectively, without getting sick. Again, the ginseng root contains coumarins (a type of phytoestrogen) which may be why some women say that it works well for them on their menopausal symptoms.

A word of caution

Studies on dong quai, black cohosh and ginseng are small and few in number. We don't have enough data yet to indicate the effects of taking these herbs or herbal supplements for the long term. Their safety and effectiveness for use during menopause is not yet established.

Evening primrose oil

Evening primrose oil is used by some women for treating menopausal symptoms. Small trials on evening primrose oil were conducted in 1998 by the Natural Therapies Unit at the Sydney Menopause Centre but they found no significant effects on menopausal symptoms. More work is needed.

St John's wort

St John's wort, *Hypericum perforatum*, is an interesting herb that is currently receiving a lot of attention. It appears that St John's wort has its main effect in the areas of depression, moods and what are called affective symptoms (those symptoms that you feel rather than see). The first report of a large-scale, well controlled trial of St John's wort has shown that it is not effective for treatment of major depressive disorder.[5] It may have a beneficial effect on mild depression.

Complementary therapies and menopausal symptoms

What may help:
- ✓ dietary phytoestrogens
- ✓ phytoestrogen supplements (isoflavonoids 40–160 mg per day)
- ✓ black cohosh
- ✓ topical progesterone cream

What probably won't help:
- ✗ evening primrose oil
- ✗ dong quai
- ✗ ginseng

There is insufficient evidence at the moment about the use of St John's wort and its recommendation for use in depression should wait until larger and longer research trials are conducted. St John's wort may also interact with some medication so, if you are taking prescription drugs, discuss the herb with your doctor before using it.

Summary of Step 5

In the area of complementary medicines for the menopause, we must take into account the fact that all these areas require further trials and investigations before any conclusive statements can be made. The evidence to date suggests that phytoestrogens, black cohosh and topical progesterone creams may work, while evening primrose oil, dong quai and ginseng probably do not work.

Questions and answers

Q. *I have been having mild hot flushes and I do not want to take HRT. Are there any alternatives?*

A. Yes, there are a number of alternatives you might want to try. You could increase the phytoestrogen content in your diet and increase your exercise (see Steps 2 and 3) to help relieve your flushes. Alternatively, try black cohosh (available from herbalists) or buying a phytoestrogen supplement such as Novogen from your pharmacy. Remember, though, to discuss these alternatives with your doctor to check if they clash with other medications you are taking.

Q. *I would like to take natural progesterone. What is the most effective way of applying it?*

A. Natural progesterone should be applied to any area of the skin that is thin, such as around the breast and chest area, so that absorption through the skin is increased. It can take up to three months to work, so if you decide to use this option, it is best to give it a few months' trial.

Q. *I have many friends who say that wild yam cream and natural progesterone are the same substance. Is this true?*

A. Wild yam cream is one of the most popular complementary therapies used by menopausal women. It does not contain natural progesterone, but it does contain a type of phytoestrogen which is found naturally in wild yams and soy beans. The effects that women may receive from taking wild yams are most likely due to the increased levels of phytoestrogens. Taking wild yams, however, will not increase your progesterone levels.

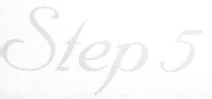

Step 5

Step **6**

Putting it into
practice

Hope is most powerful when backed up by action.

R. Gilbert, *Bits and Pieces*, 1999

Hope is a powerful thing. If we approach menopause and beyond with hope rather than confusion and despair, we can make it work for us instead of against us. And hope that is supported by informed action is the most powerful force of all.

We have worked through the six steps containing the information that will make your menopause terrific. We would now like to share with you the means by which you can make it happen and implement these steps into your life— the sixth and final step of *The Menopause Made Simple Program.*

You may have thought you were near the end of the book, but really we are just at the beginning of the journey. You are about to undertake a 12-week program that will set in place such positive exercise, eating and empowering habits that you will never be able to turn back.

First, however, you have a task to do—go out and buy something you like to congratulate yourself on getting this far and to mark the beginning of our journey together. This special thing need not be expensive, just something that makes you feel good. Perhaps the ingredients for your favourite meal or a bunch of those beautiful tulips that have just come into bloom? Or why not buy that lovely gold frame for that special picture you want to keep?

Why are you doing this? You are telling yourself that you are special and worth investing in.

18

The Menopause Made Simple Program

The greatest mistake a man (woman) can ever make is to sacrifice health for any other advantage.

Arthur Schopenhauer

You now have all the information you need to understand menopause, how it might affect you and what you can do to manage it. The next and most important step is to move forward and put these strategies into place.

The 12-week program in the next chapter takes you through each step, giving you daily or weekly focus points to ease your journey. We pull all the information together and present it as an easy-to-follow plan. Using this time frame, you can introduce the various components and ideas and bring them into your life slowly over 12 weeks. The steps build on each other and help you to make healthy lifestyle changes.

Make sure you give yourself plenty of self-encouragement. Remind yourself daily how well you are doing and focus on the aspects that are going well. You can achieve your goals by deciding that this program is an important priority in your life for the next 12 weeks. As you start making one simple lifestyle change and feel the benefits of it, you will be encouraged to continue. It is a good feeling when you realise that you have the ability to change your life and that you can control your destiny by the choices you make.

As we said earlier, the kind of menopause you experience seems to be related to what you expect it to be. If you expect menopause to be a time of doom and gloom, then most likely you will experience a range of emotional and physical symptoms that correlates with that expectation. If you see menopause as a positive new stage in your life, when your body is adjusting to changes in hormone levels, then the chances are you will sail through it with vibrance and enthusiasm.

Having a healthy body and mind will allow you to make the most of this time of your life. Embark on the next 12 weeks knowing that you will never look back.

Taking the steps

Let's look at the six steps that you can follow to make your transition through menopause smooth and fulfilling.

- Step 1—Seek out reliable health information
- Step 2—Eat a healthy diet during menopause
- Step 3—Exercise regularly during menopause
- Step 4—Determine whether HRT is for you
- Step 5—Consider complementary therapies
- Step 6—Put it into practice.

In Step 1, *Health information*, we provided you with the latest information about menopause. We want you to be armed with the correct, non-biased information so you can make choices that suit you. You are an individual and only you know what is right for you. Understanding menopause takes the uncertainty out of what you can expect and puts you in the driver's seat.

Taking Step 2, *Eating for menopause*, is important. No matter what else you do, it is essential to eat a healthy and nutritious diet. You cannot expect to reap rewards if you are consuming a diet of processed foods high in saturated fats, sugar and salt. You are what you eat. The quality of food that you consume each day is one of the fundamental influences over how your body functions.

Exercise is important at all stages of our lives, but the benefits you will receive from regular exercise during menopause are immeasurable. In Step 3, *Exercising for menopause*, we looked at the types of exercise that are most beneficial and at how you can introduce them into your life. Don't underestimate exercise. It will help you to maintain strong bones, strengthen muscles, preserve balance, maintain your weight, minimise lifestyle diseases and increase your confidence and self-esteem.

In Steps 4 and 5, we looked at the options for taking HRT, in the short and long term, and at the alternatives available if you decide against HRT.

How to start the program

In Step 6 we look at how to implement this program. First, make a photocopy of the final chapter of this book—the journal. Keep it in a folder and record your progress. This is your guide to take you step by step each day to put into practice the information that you have gained. Choose the date on which you will start the program—ideally a Monday—and mark it on the calendar. Arm yourself with the journal and let's go.

Staying positive

It is important when doing a program like this to stay positive. Don't worry if you miss a day—the important thing is to cover the general concepts and build them into your everyday life. We don't achieve success the first time we try. Stay focused on the reasons that you want to work through the program—a stronger, healthier more vibrant you, a woman in control of her own menopause.

Measuring your success

Throughout the program there are small goals to achieve along the way, together with ideas on how to measure how well you are doing. It is a good idea to note in your journal how you are feeling before you start the program. Repeat this exercise once each month and you will be surprised at how much you have achieved in four weeks. If you stick with the program for 12 weeks, you will be amazed at how fabulous and in control you feel. Remember, if you can adopt these new lifestyle habits over 12 weeks, you are very likely to continue them for the rest of your life.

How to use the journal

The first two weeks of the program are outlined daily in the journal. The next six weeks are broken down weekly, and the last month, fortnightly. This guides you through the program gradually, giving you more flexibility as you become confident.

On page 214 we have outlined a sample you can use to record your exercise progress. You can photocopy this or use a notebook.

After the program

When the 12 weeks are over, you will be ready to continue your new positive menopausal behaviours for the rest of your menopause and indeed for the rest of your life. All women go through this journey at some stage; our experience and wisdom can be passed on to future generations of women to ensure that menopause is a rewarding journey and that they become vibrant and exceptional older women. Enjoy the journey—we have loved taking part of it with you!

Chapter 19

The Menopause Made Simple Program Journal

Live your life each day as you would climb a mountain. An occasional glance towards the summit keeps the goal in mind, but many beautiful scenes are to be observed from each new vantage point. Climb slowly, steadily, enjoying each passing moment. The view from the summit will serve as a fitting climax for the journey.

Harold V. Melchert

Week 1 / Day 1   **Date:** _____

> *Motivation is what gets you started.*
> *Habit is what keeps you going.*
> R. Gilbert, *Bits and Pieces*, 1999

- Think about maintaining a positive attitude throughout the day. You can change the way you feel about things by adjusting your perspective on life. Focus on what you *have*, not on what you don't have. In her book *Simple Abundance*, Sara Ban Breathnach encourages us each day to write down five things that we are grateful for. This exercise immediately forces us to look at the positives in our lives. Her book is an excellent companion that can help lead you to 'a happier, more fulfilling and contented way of life'.

- Buy yourself a bunch of flowers that you really like. Put them in a place where you will see them frequently. If you are at work, place them on your desk and enjoy the stimulation you receive to your senses every time you look at them.

- Think about how much water you are drinking. If you don't have a water bottle invest in one to have at work or to take with you when you go out. Keep a jug of water in the fridge with sliced lemon or lime. Try to build up to eight glasses of water a day by the end of the week. Remember—your body will adjust to the increase in fluids and regulate itself.

Things I feel happy about:

1. _____

_____

_____

2. _____

_____

_____

3. _____

_____

_____

Things I would like to improve on:

1. _____

_____

_____

2. _____

_____

_____

3. _____

_____

_____

Week 1 / Day 2   **Date:** _____

- Try to have three different pieces of fruit today. By increasing the amount of fruit you eat you will usually cut down on other types of higher-fat snacks. Of course, you will benefit from the extra vitamins and phytoestrogens that fruit contains. Try to think about variety— make up a bowl of fruit salad and include fruits you wouldn't normally eat.

Fruit I ate today:

1. _____

2. _____

3. _____

- Keep the focus on your water intake.
- Decide what time of the day best suits you to start walking tomorrow:
    - Organise anything you need to make it happen.
    - Work out the best time of the day for you to walk.
    - Iron clothes the night before.
    - Make lunches before you go to bed.
    - If you are walking in the morning, lay out your walking clothes and shoes.
    - Set the alarm earlier.

Today I felt (record your feelings, moods, thoughts):

_____

_____

_____

_____

_____

_____

_____

_____

_____

_____

_____

_____

_____

_____

_____

_____

_____

_____

_____

_____

_____

_____

Week 1 / Day 3   Date: _____

Start walking. Use today to determine for how long you can walk comfortably. It may be ten minutes or maybe 30 minutes. This will be an individual starting point. The average will probably be 15–20 minutes. Remember to walk tall, eyes forward, not down. Start on a fairly flat area until you build up your fitness.

Today I walked for _____ minutes.

My walk felt:
- ❏ *Very easy*—I felt like I didn't have to exert myself at all.
- ❏ *Easy*—I could notice I was walking but little effort was required.
- ❏ *Moderate*—I could feel my heart beating faster than normal, but I would have had no problem having a conversation.
- ❏ *Hard*—I felt I was puffing. And I started to tire towards the end.
- ❏ *Very hard*—I had difficulty continuing and would not have been able to hold a conversation.

When you initially start walking, aim to be working at the moderate intensity level. This will give your body a chance to get used to the exercise.

If you felt the intensity was lower than moderate, you need to increase the pace that you walk at.

Don't forget to drink lots of water when you return, and give yourself a big pat on the back for making a start.

Well done—you have started a healthy lifestyle activity that can reduce your risk of heart disease and osteoporosis and help to reduce your weight.

Week 1 / Day 4   Date: _____

Set aside half an hour to clean out the fridge and pantry. Be ruthless and get rid of anything that is out of date, or not going to contribute to your healthy lifestyle. High-fat foods and snacks like biscuits and chips are better not left in the pantry on a regular basis. That doesn't mean you can't have occasional treats—it's the balanced approach that will bring you long-term success.

There is something very therapeutic about sorting through our surroundings. Having an orderly pantry and fridge sets you up to see what things you need to buy.

Revise the shopping list below and add any new items that you need to include.

Suggested shopping list for the menopausal woman:
- variety of fresh fruit and vegetables
- low-fat/high-calcium milk
- low-fat soy milk
- soy and linseed bread
- low-fat/high-calcium yoghurt
- breakfast cereal containing soy (with or without linseeds)
- tinned salmon/tuna/sardines
- fresh fish
- raw mixed nuts
- packet of linseeds (to sprinkle in muffins, over cereal)
- rice/pasta
- lean red meat/chicken
- olive/canola oil.

Today I felt:

_____

_____

_____

_____

_____

_____

_____

_____

_____

_____

_____

_____

_____

_____

_____

_____

_____

_____

_____

_____

_____

_____

Week 1 / Day 5   Date: _____

- Go for your second walk today. Try to walk for the same length of time as on your first walk or if you are feeling stronger, add five minutes. Don't forget to drink plenty of water when you get back.

I walked for _____ minutes.

The intensity level of the walk was:
- ❑ Very easy
- ❑ Easy
- ❑ Moderate
- ❑ Hard
- ❑ Very hard.

Today I ate _____ pieces of fruit.

- Do a shop using the shopping list you made yesterday. You may have a few extra items this week as you are stocking the pantry, but many of these will not be weekly buys. Choose a couple of fruits or vegetables that you wouldn't normally buy, so that you start to get more variety.

Week 1 / Day 6

Date: _____

It's time to do a calcium stocktake to determine whether you are getting enough. Record what you eat today so you can determine the calcium values. This is just a guide—you don't have to weigh or measure your food.

Date:

	What I ate	Calcium content
Breakfast	_____	_____
	_____	_____
	_____	_____
	_____	_____
	_____	_____
	_____	_____
Morning tea	_____	_____
	_____	_____
	_____	_____
Lunch	_____	_____
	_____	_____
	_____	_____
	_____	_____
	_____	_____
	_____	_____
	_____	_____

	What I ate	Calcium content
Afternoon tea	_____	_____
	_____	_____
	_____	_____
Dinner	_____	_____
	_____	_____
	_____	_____
	_____	_____
	_____	_____
	_____	_____
Supper	_____	_____
	_____	_____
Other snacks	_____	_____
	_____	_____
	_____	_____
	_____	_____
Total	_____	

Put the calcium content of your food on the sheet and tally up your daily amounts (see page 50).

Compare these values with the recommended daily intakes (RDI).

- If you are taking HRT, it is 1000 mg per day.
- If you are not taking HRT, you need 1500 mg per day.

My calcium is higher/lower than my RDI. I need to increase my calcium by _____ mg per day.

If you are not getting enough calcium, you need to think about ways to increase it.

- Use calcium-fortified milks. They will give you an extra 140 mg of calcium per every 250 ml glass of milk.
- Add a yoghurt each day for a morning or afternoon snack.
- Have a glass of milk before you go to bed.
- Include cereal for breakfast a few times a week. You will get about 300 mg of calcium from the milk used.
- Make a tasty milkshake by blending a banana and skim milk—great for an afternoon snack. (Try other fruits such as strawberries or mangoes.)
- Have a glass of soy milk each day (ensure that it has added calcium). The phytoestrogens it contains are as valuable as the calcium.

Week 1 / Day 7   Date: _____

On Sunday it is a good idea to plan your exercise for the following week. If day 7 does not fall on a Sunday replan it so it does. Pull out your diary or weekly organiser sheet (see below) and write in the days that you plan to exercise next week. This will help you work around any other activities that may be on. Writing it down is a good way of committing yourself even more.

Time	Mon	Tue	Wed	Thurs	Fri	Sat	Sun

Write down the times that suit you in the left-hand column (see example opposite). Planning for the week ahead allows you to adjust your schedule. For example, if you have a dinner on the night before you normally walk that you know will go late, then you can move your walk to another day.

Time	Mon	Tue	Wed	Thurs	Fri	Sat	Sun
6–7 am	Walk			Walk			
7–9 am							
9–5 pm							Walk
5–6 pm							
6–7 pm		Dinner with Susan					
7–8 pm						Movies	
8–10 pm							

Exercise

Take a walk today. Don't forget to look around and enjoy your surround-ings. Take in the trees, watch the clouds and listen to the birds.

I walked for _____ minutes today and the intensity level was _____.

Well done! You have taken some important steps towards living a healthier lifestyle.

This week I have:

- started exercising
- increased the amount of water I drink each day
- eaten more fruit
- made sure I am getting enough calcium
- stocked the fridge and pantry with healthy and nutritious food
- planned my exercise for next week.

Week 2 / Day 1   Date: _____

Do a checklist of your waterworks system.

Do you have any of the following?

- ❏   Leakage when you sneeze, cough or laugh
- ❏   A feeling of urgency to pass urine
- ❏   The need to go to the toilet frequently.

If you have any of these symptoms that we discussed in Step 3, it is wise to follow up with a qualified health professional. Visit your general practitioner first, who will rule out the possibility that these symptoms are caused by urinary tract infections. They can then refer you to a specialist health nurse or physiotherapist specialising in urinary incontinence.

Even if you don't have any of these symptoms it is still important for you to start doing pelvic floor exercises to prevent any problems in the future. Re-read Chapter 11 on pelvic floor exercises and start doing the exercise plan (page 106) today.

Today I feel happy about:

1. _____

_____

_____

_____

_____

_____

_____

2. _____

_____

_____

_____

_____

_____

_____

3. _____

_____

_____

_____

_____

_____

_____

Week 2 / Day 2

Date: _____

Phytoestrogens—you know what they are and where you can get them, but are you getting enough? Write down your food intake today and check the approximate amount of phytoestrogens you are getting.

	What I ate	Phytoestrogen content
Breakfast	_____	_____
	_____	_____
	_____	_____
Morning tea	_____	_____
	_____	_____
	_____	_____
Lunch	_____	_____
	_____	_____
	_____	_____
Afternoon tea	_____	_____
	_____	_____
	_____	_____
Dinner	_____	_____
	_____	_____
	_____	_____

	What I ate	Phytoestrogen content
Supper	_____	_____
	_____	_____
Other snacks	_____	_____
	_____	_____
Total	_____	_____

- 300 ml serving of soy milk contains about 15–20 mg of phytoestrogens.
- 55 g of tofu contains about 35–40 mg of phytoestrogens.
- Two slices of soy and linseed bread contains about 22 mg of phytoestrogens.
- 45 g serving of soy breakfast cereal contains about 36 mg of phytoestrogens.

We are aiming for 45–60 mg per day. If you are falling short of this amount here are some easy ways to increase the phytoestrogens in your diet on a regular basis:

- glass of soy milk
- soy and linseed bread
- soy breakfast cereal with a sprinkle of linseeds
- fresh fruit and vegetables.

Week 2 / Day 3

Date: _____

Go for your walk but, today, add some stretches when you have finished. It should only take you an extra five minutes to perform the stretches outlined in Chapter 10 (page 100).

- hamstring
- quadricep
- gluteals
- shoulder
- chest.

Remember:

- Stretch in a slow and controlled manner.
- Avoid bouncy, ballistic movements.
- Hold each stretch for 15–20 seconds, alternating each side.
- Repeat three to four times on each side.

As you breathe out, relax and move deeper into the stretch. Include these stretches after each walk.

Exercise	Time
Walk	_____ minutes
Stretches	❑ (tick)

Try to drink eight glasses of water today.

Week 2 / Day 4   **Date:** _____

Things work out best for those who make the
best of the way things work out.

Think about how stress affects your life. Take time to reflect on whether you feel you have high, medium or low stress levels.

I feel my stress levels are:
❑ low
❑ medium
❑ high

Sometimes low stress levels can be just as difficult to cope with as high stress levels. Not having enough in your life to keep you active and stimulated can cause you stress without you realising it. Try to identify the causes of your stress and think about ways of minimising the feelings.

The areas that cause stress in my life relate to:
❑ health
❑ spouse
❑ children
❑ caring for parents
❑ work pressures
❑ finances
❑ other _____.

We must give ourselves time to regenerate our mind and body, whether through exercise, personal time or a positive attitude. If we don't learn how to control the stress in our lives it can lead to health problems in the future.

Write down three things that you can do to improve the stress in your life:

1. _____

_____

2. _____

_____

3. _____

_____

Consider using some of these stress management strategies:

- yoga
- relaxation and/or meditation
- carving out time for yourself
- tai chi
- counselling and support.

Stress comes from our perceptions of events rather than the events themselves. Remind yourself frequently: 'I can control my stress.'

Week 2 / Day 5   **Date:** _____

*Friendship is like a bank account. You can't continue to
draw on it without making deposits.*

- Contact a friend you haven't spoken to in a while and rekindle the friendship.
- Go for a walk and do the stretches.
- While you are doing your stretches, practise the paced respiration for controlling hot flushes.

Breathe in for five seconds, then slowly breathe out for five seconds. Now try to make the breath last a little longer. Breathe in for seven seconds, breathe out for seven seconds. Practise this controlled breathing as you do the stretches. As soon as you feel a hot flush beginning, start paced respirations. Sometimes, a hot flush will begin with a tingling sensation in your fingers and toes. Continue controlled breathing until the flush is over.

If you are not experiencing hot flushes then rejoice and enjoy the relaxed feeling you will experience from controlled breathing.

Exercise	Time
Walk	_____ minutes
Stretches	❑ (tick)

Where I am doing well:

_____

_____

_____

_____

_____

_____

_____

_____

Where I can improve on:

_____

_____

_____

_____

_____

_____

_____

Week 2 / Day 6   Date: _____

Find a new recipe and try something you wouldn't normally cook. Take the time to set the table with candles and flowers. Turn off the TV, open a bottle of wine and enjoy good company.

A new recipe:

_____

_____

_____

_____

_____

_____

_____

_____

_____

_____

_____

_____

_____

_____

_____

_____

_____

Week 2 / Day 7   **Date:** _____

Prepare your weekly plan for next week.

- In your organiser or diary work out your days for exercising.
- Set yourself a goal you would like to accomplish for next week. It might be to do with work, personal health or simply to smile more. Keep it simple but specific, and write it down.

Next week I would like to achieve:

_____

_____

_____

_____

_____

- If you smoke, then make it your goal to stop. This will be the best thing you will ever do for yourself. Make a date to stop, seek advice from your doctor or pharmacist and enlist the support of family and friends.
- Increase your walking time by five to ten minutes.
- Think about meeting a friend to walk with next week.

Exercise	Time
Walk	_____ minutes
Stretching	❏ (tick)

Week 3 / Day 1   Date: _____

Make a checklist of your health and menopausal symptoms to determine what options for HRT or alternative therapies suit you best.

Health checklist	
Family history	*Details*
❑ Heart disease	_____
❑ High blood pressure	_____
❑ High cholesterol	_____
❑ Osteoporosis	_____
Personal history	*Details*
❑ Heart disease	_____
❑ High blood pressure	_____
❑ High cholesterol	_____
❑ Osteoporosis	_____
❑ Arthritis	_____
❑ Cigarette smoking	_____
How many per day?	_____
❑ Physical inactivity	_____
❑ Overweight/obesity	_____
❑ Diabetes	_____
❑ Asthma	_____
❑ Poor dietary practices	_____
❑ Muscle pains	_____
❑ Joint pain	_____
❑ Other	_____

Do you experience any of these on a regular basis?

❑ Hot flushes   ❑ Headaches

❑ Night sweats   ❑ Insomnia

❑ Vaginal irritation or dryness   ❑ Lack of energy

❑ Irregular periods   ❑ Fluid retention

❑ Depression   ❑ Backache

❑ Nervous tension   ❑ Difficulty in concentration

❑ Palpitations   ❑ Dizzy spells

Make an appointment to see your doctor. Take along the checklist so that you have all the information the doctor will require.

Do you need to ask about:

❑ A cholesterol check?

❑ A pap smear?

❑ A breast examination and/or mammogram?

❑ Bone density scan?

❑ HRT?

❑ Complementary therapies?

❑ Exercise (you may have problems with your neck, back, arthritis etc.)?

Remember, you have all the information you need to decide what options are best for you.

• Continue walking three times a week, slowly increasing the time to reach 30 minutes. Record your progress in an exercise diary (see page 214).

Week 4   Week beginning: _____

Well done—you have been exercising regularly for three weeks now and it is time to introduce some strength training into your program.

Decide where you will do your strength training, at home or in a fitness centre. Do you need help from a fitness trainer or will you follow the program outlined in this book? Aim to do strength exercises twice a week.

If you decide to go to a fitness centre, look in the phone book for local centres. Find out services and prices over the phone and then visit the ones that seem suitable. Ask whether a program is provided for you and whether an instructor will show you how to do the exercises.

If you plan to do strength training at home, find an area that you can use and decide on a suitable time. You might like to add the exercises at the end of your walk. (Allow an hour to do a 30-minute walk, strength exercises and stretching.) If this doesn't work, set two times in your organiser that fit in.

If you decide to follow the program in this book, begin with Program I (page 87) twice a week—exercises without equipment:

- squats
- lunges
- modified pushups
- seated tricep dips
- abdominals and pelvic floor
- lower back
- stretches.

Do two sets of eight to ten repetitions.

Think about the technique you are using. Don't try to rush.

- Aim for slow, controlled movement.
- It is normal to feel some muscle soreness for the first few weeks. Your muscles are being used in a new way. Stretching will help to minimise and relieve the soreness.
- Start slowly and build up gradually.

Record your progress in the exercise diary.

Week 5   Week beginning: _____

Strong Bones Week

Prevention of osteoporosis is extremely important. If you don't put lifestyle strategies into place now to minimise bone loss your bones won't last the distance. This week ensure that you are doing everything you can to keep your bones strong and healthy for the rest of your life.

Strong bones depend on:

- Maximising peak bone density in childhood and adolescence.
- Maintaining bone density throughout adult life.

We have talked about *peak bone density* and how the level of bone density you achieve during this important developmental stage will set you up for life. Peak bone mass is usually achieved in mid- to late-twenties, so the years leading up to this period will determine the maximum amount of your bone density. Take the time to talk to daughters, nieces and friends that fall into this age group and educate them on how crucial a time it is for determining peak bone density. You could be contributing to a healthier quality of life for them in their senior years.

To maintain bone density throughout life you should:

- consume a healthy diet with adequate calcium content (1000 mg HRT, 1500 mg without HRT)
- ensure sufficient intake of vitamin D (10–15 minutes of sunshine daily)
- do regular weight-bearing exercise
- minimise alcohol intake
- not smoke.

How many of the healthy lifestyle behaviours have you put into place to ensure strong healthy bones for life?

Refer back to the tips on preventing osteoporosis on page 32.

Week 6   **Week beginning:** _____

- Pamper yourself! Book a massage or facial to indulge yourself. If that's not a viable option, set aside some time to give yourself a facial. Make it feel special—put on some music, light some candles and sit in the bath with a glass of wine.
- Make sure that you are including all the healthy eating principles in your diet.

Each day I am:

	Always	Sometimes	Never
Drinking eight glasses of water	❑	❑	❑
Eating at least two pieces of fruit	❑	❑	❑
Having three servings or more of vegetables	❑	❑	❑
Eating wholegrain breads, cereals, rice and pastas	❑	❑	❑
Using monounsaturated oil for cooking			
(i.e. canola or olive oil)	❑	❑	❑
Minimising the amount of fat in my diet	❑	❑	❑
Having less than three cups of coffee	❑	❑	❑
Not adding extra salt to my food	❑	❑	❑
Not having more than two alcoholic drinks	❑	❑	❑
Having three to four servings of calcium	❑	❑	❑
Eating foods that are high in phytoestrogens	❑	❑	❑
(e.g. soy, linseeds, tofu)	❑	❑	❑

The areas I am doing well in with my diet are:

_____

_____

_____

_____

_____

_____

_____

_____

_____

The areas I need to focus on in my diet are:

_____

_____

_____

_____

_____

_____

_____

_____

_____

_____

Week 7   **Week beginning:** _____

Healthy Heart Week

Having a healthy heart is crucial to our everyday life. If our heart is not working properly nothing else matters.

Did you know that:

1. Coronary heart disease is the number one cause of death in the Western world?

2. One-third of all heart attacks end in death (one-half of all first attacks)?

3. Nearly twice as many people die from heart disease as from all kinds of cancer?

4. Sometimes heart disease presents no warning symptoms (Griggs, 1990).

This week ensure that you are living a life that will help your heart to stay healthy. These are the risk factors you can control:

- *Blood pressure.* Check it regularly—if you have high blood pressure ensure that it is managed through either medication or diet and exercise.

- *Cholesterol levels.* Regular checks can ensure that it is kept at healthy levels.

- *Smoking.* If you haven't already stopped, think long and hard about how you can do this for yourself.

- *Stress.* Know where your stress comes from and try to minimise the effect that it has your life.

- *Weight control.* Keep your weight at a healthy level.

There are plenty of things you can do to protect your heart.

- Have a healthy diet that is:
  - low in saturated fats
  - high in unsaturated fats (eat fish two to three times a week)
  - high in fruit and vegetables (aim for seven servings a day)
  - high in fibre-rich foods.
- Do regular cardiovascular or aerobic exercise.
- Control your stress and maintain a positive mental attitude.

Refer back to the tips for preventing cardiovascular disease on page 28.

I know that my heart is affected by the way I live my life.
By looking after my mind and body I am keeping my heart
healthy and strong.

Week 8   **Week beginning:** _____

- Revisit the health checklist (page 198) and rate your menopausal symptoms again. Have any of them improved?

- Check your intensity level when you are walking. You might have started with a level that felt 'moderate' but now you need to increase your walking pace so that it feels 'hard'. That means that you are puffing and starting to tire towards the end of the walk. You are now fitter and can cope with an increase in intensity.

My walk felt:

❑ *Very easy*—I felt I didn't have to exert myself at all.

❑ *Easy*—I could notice I was walking but little effort was required.

❑ *Moderate*—I could feel my heart beating faster than normal, but I would have had no problem having a conversation.

❑ *Hard*—I felt I was puffing, and I started to tire towards the end.

❑ *Very hard*—I had difficulty continuing and would not have been able to hold a conversation.

Week 9   Week beginning: _____

Cancer Prevention Week

Many people are terrified of the 'C' word. We have all known or heard of someone who was struck down prematurely by cancer. There are so many different types of cancer and each one is affected by different factors. However, there are lifestyle habits that have been associated with low cancer risk. This week, focus on ensuring that your lifestyle is aimed at preventing cancer.

These lifestyle behaviours include:
- Regular exercise
- A diet with:
  - plenty of fresh fruit, vegetables and wholegrain foods
  - a small amount of fat
  - low intake of red meat and more fish
  - low intake of processed foods
  - high intake of phytoestrogens
- No smoking
- Moderate alcohol consumption
- Weight control
- Regular use of suncreen
- Managed stress levels
- Regular medical checkups
- Reporting any unusual bleeding, discharge or lumps.

Refer back to page 34 for tips on preventing breast cancer.

I can control my risk of cancer.
I have a balanced lifestyle that is healthy and enjoyable.

Week 10   **Week beginning:** _____

- Start a new hobby or interest. Think about what you have always wanted to do. Maybe it's pottery, yoga, learning a language, golf, quilting or needlework. Look for a course or group you can join.

I would like to start: _____

- Congratulations! You have been doing your strength training exercises for six weeks. You should be starting to feel a little stronger. You may already feel that your balance and flexibility have improved. If you are doing your exercises at home, using Program 1, you might like to think about investing in some dumbbells that will allow you to take your program to another level. So far, you have been using your own body as a resistance—now you are strong enough to add some extra weight.

    At this stage you could consider purchasing a pair each of 2, 3 and 4 kg weights. Most exercise supply stores stock these, or you could look in the classifieds for second-hand weights. An alternative to set dumbbells is the kind that allow you to change the weight. They consist of a handle with weighted plates that can be slid on and off to adjust the weight. They might be a little more expensive to start with, but they allow you to increase the weight without purchasing several pairs of dumbbells. The most weight you will probably ever need, no matter how long you have been training, is 10 kg.

Store your dumbbells in a bag or box so they are not left lying around for you or someone else to trip over. When doing strength training, focus on the muscle you are using and try to visualise it doing the work.

Program 2—Exercises with dumbbells (do two sets of eight to ten repetitions). Refer to Chapter 10.

- squats
- lunges
- modified pushups
- shoulder press
- tricep extension
- abdominals and pelvic floor
- lower back
- stretches.

Squats and lunges remain the same, but you will add some weights to hold.

Abdominals, pelvic floor, lower back and stretches continue as before.

Don't forget to record your progress in your exercise diary.

Week 12 **Week beginning:** _____

Use this week to reflect on the balance of your life. Think of how much time and energy is devoted to the different areas of your life. Is one part of your life absorbing much more of your energy than the others?

My life:

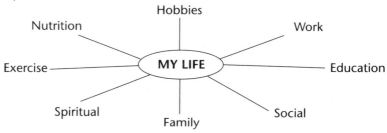

Think of ways and activities you can do to lead a more balanced life.

1. _____

   _____

2. _____

   _____

3. _____

   _____

Goal setting helps you to organise and prioritise your life. Try to set some goals for yourself for the following time frames. Keep them achievable and realistic. These are your goals and you do not need to show them to anyone—so be honest with yourself!

In one month I would like to: _____

_____

_____

Six months: _____

_____

_____

One year: _____

_____

_____

Five years: _____

_____

_____

Shoot for the moon ... even if you miss, you'll be among the stars.

Changing your life takes time. We are talking about changing habits that you have probably had for many years. But persevere—if you can do something for 28 days you have formed a new habit. Remember that you have the controls: accept your circumstances, whatever they may be, and move forward.

Exercise diary

Date: _____

❑ Walking _____ minutes

❑ Strength training

Exercise	Repetitions	Sets	Weight
Abdominals			
Pelvic floor			
Lower back			

❑ Stretching

Comments: _____

_____

_____

Long-term studies into HRT use

The Women's Health Initiative

One of the largest studies to date, the Women's Health Initiative (WHI), funded by US$625 million, has been designed to look at the effects on cardiovascular disease, cancer and osteoporosis of HRT, diet, dietary supplements, exercise and the cessation of smoking. The final results are due in 2008.

If you want to know more about this study, and the results to date, visit the website at www.nhlbi.nih.gov/whi/index.html

The Postmenopausal Estrogen/Progestin Intervention (PEPI) Trial

This large three-year study has been completed. It explored a number of issues related to HRT. Results confirmed that HRT had improved bone preservation, blood lipid levels, the cardiovascular system and the endometrium. Questions on its association with breast cancer risk and the long-term effects of HRT are still unconfirmed.

More information about this study can be found at www.ama-assn.org/special/womh/library/readroom/vol_280a/joc80678.htm

The Million Women Study

In the UK, research involving the recruitment of one million menopausal and postmenopausal women was initiated in 1997 to help determine whether HRT actually increases the risk of developing breast cancer.

Visit the website at www.icnet.uk/research/studies/mws/index2.html

The Women's International Study of long Duration Oestrogen after Menopause (WISDOM)

The WISDOM study is designed to look at the risks and benefits of hormone replacement therapy in (postmenopausal) women. The study will commence in 2002 and last for ten years. It will look at 34 000 postmenopausal women in 14 countries, including Australia. Initial results are expected in the year 2012.

You can find out more about this study at www.pslgroup.com/dg/de66.htm

The Heart and Estrogen–progestin Replacement Study (HERS)

This study aims to determine the differences in outcomes of women who take HRT and women who have never taken HRT. The HERS study has reported some of the most significant results to date on the effects of HRT on the cardiovascular system.

More information can be found at www.med.stanford.edu/fm/?/school/scrdp/research/studies/&women_hers2.html

Endnotes

Step 1: Health information

1 Fu, 2000
2 Dennerstein et al., 1993; Avis & McKinlay, 1991
3 Anderson, 1999
4 Hammar et al., 1990
5 Freedman & Woodward, 1992
6 Gordon, 1976
7 Punyahotra et al., 1997
8 Van Hall et al., 1994
9 Law, 1991
10 Lindsay et al., 1980
11 NBCC, 1999

Step 2: Eating for menopause

1 Knight et al., 1996
2 Knight et al., 1996
3 Knight et al., 1996
4 Aldercreutz et al., 1995
5 Knight et al., 1996

Step 3: Exercising for menopause

1 Dennerstein et al., 1993

Step 4: Hormone replacement therapy

1 NHMRC, 1999
2 Clinical Synthesis Conference, 1999
3 Sturdee, 1997
4 Ballinger, 1990
5 Beral et al., 1999; WHO, 1996; International Agency for Research on Cancer, 1999; Collaborative Group on Hormonal Factors in Breast Cancer, 1997; Clinical Synthesis Conference, 1999
6 Beral et al., 1999
7 WHO, 1996; Beral et al., 1999
8 Lindsay, 1988
9 Hulley et al., 1998
10 Hulley et al., 1998; Stewart, 1998
11 IMS, 2000

Step 5: Alternatives to HRT

1 McLennan et al., 1996
2 Anderson, 1999
3 Knight et al., 1996
4 Husband, 2001
5 Shelton, 2001

Further reading

Greene, B. & Winfrey, O. *Make the Connection: Ten Steps to a Better Body and a Better Life*, Century Books, 1996

Nelson, M. & Wernick, S. *Strong Women Stay Slim*, Thomas C. Lothian, 1998

Nelson, M. & Wernick, S. *Strong Women Stay Young*, Thomas C. Lothian, 1997

Stewart, M. *The Phyto Factor: The Exciting New Medical Breakthrough on the Natural Power of Phytoestrogen-Rich Foods*, Hodder & Stoughton, 1998

Bibliography

Aldercreutz, H., Goldin, B.R., Gorbach, S.L. 'Soybean phytoestrogen intake and cancer risk', *Journal of Nutrition*, 1995, 125: 757–770

Aldercreutz, H., Mazur, W. 'Phyto-oestrogens and Western diseases', *Annals of Medicine*, 1997, 29: 95–100

Aldercreutz, H., Honjo H., Higashi, A. et al. 'Urinary excretion of lignans and isoflavonoid phytoestrogens in Japanese men and women consuming a traditional Japanese diet', *American Journal of Clinical Nutrition*, 1991, 54:1093–1100

American Cancer Society, 'Long-term estrogens increase ovarian cancer mortality risk', *JAMA*, 2001, 285:1460–1465

Anderson, D. 'Responses to the Menopause: Hormone Replacement Therapy and Alternatives', unpublished PhD thesis, University of Queensland, 1999

Avis, N.E. 'Women's perceptions of the menopause', *European Menopause Journal*, 1996, 3(2): 80–84

Avis, N.E., McKinlay, S.M. 'A longitudinal analysis of women's attitudes toward the menopause: results from the Massachusetts Women's Health Study', *Maturitas*, 1991, 13(1): 65–79

Ballinger, C.B. 'Psychiatric aspects of the menopause', *British Journal of Psychiatry*, 1990, 156, 773–787

Beral, V., Banks, E., Reeves, G., & Appleby, P. 'Use of HRT and the subsequent risk of cancer', *Journal of Epidemiology and Biostatistics*, 1999, 4(3):191–215

Braun, K. 'Complementary medicine', *Health Journey*, Women's Health Queensland Wide, 1999, Summer

Building Better Bones Kit, Queensland Dairy Authority, 1997

Caplan, G.A., Ward, J. A. & Lord, S.R. 'The benefits of exercise in postmenopausal women', *Australian Journal of Public Health* 17, no. 1 (March 1993): 23–6

Chirawatkul, S., Manderson, L. 'Perceptions of menopause in northeast Thailand: contested meaning and practice', *Social Science Medicine*, 1994, 4: 214–220

Chompootweep, S., Tankeyoon, M., Yamarat, K., Poomsuwan, P., Dusitsin, N. 'The menopausal age and climacteric complaints in Thai women in Bangkok', *Maturitas*, 1993, Jul, 17(1), 63–71

Clinical Synthesis Conference on HRT, 'Hormone replacement therapy', *Lancet*, July, 1999: 354

Colemen, E. Siberian Ginseng Healthcare Reality Check FAQ Sheet, 2001–04–20, www.hcrc.org/faqs/sibgen.html

Collaborative Group on Hormonal Factors in Breast Cancer. 'Breast cancer and hormone replacement therapy: collaborative reanalysis of data from 51 epidemiological studies of 52 705 women with breast cancer and 108 411 women without breast cancer', *Lancet* 1997, 350:1047–59

Coope, J. 'Hormonal and non-hormonal interventions for menopausal symptoms', *Maturitas*, 1996, 23:159–168

Cummings, S,R., Cauley, J.A., Palermo, I. et al. 'Racial differences in hip axis lengths might explain racial differences in rates of hip fracture'. (Study of Osteoporotic Fractures Research Group), *Osteoporosis Int*, 1994 July, 4(4): 226–9

Dalsky, G.P. et al. 'Weight-bearing exercise training and lumbar bone mineral content in postmenopausal women, *Annals of Internal Medicine*, 108, no. 6 (June 1988): 824–8.

Delmas, P.D. 'HRT in the prevention and treatment of osteoporosis', *Journal of Epidemiology and Biostatistics*, 1999, vol 4, no 3: 155–163

Dennerstein, L., Lehert, P., Burger, H. & Dudley, E. 'Mood and sexuality', *Australasian Menopause Society Annual Congress Conference Program*, Oct. 1998

Dennerstein, L., Smith, A., Morse, C., Burger, H., Green, A., Hopper, J., & Ryan, M. 'Menopausal symptoms in Australian women', Key Centre for Women's Health in Society, Carlton, Vic. *Medical Journal of Australia*, 1993, Aug. 16, 159(4): 232–6

Eden, J. 'New options: phytoestrogens, natural progesterone', *Australasian Menopause Society Annual Congress Conference Program*, Oct. 1998

Ettinger, B., Genant, H.K., Cann, C.E. 'Postmenopausal bone loss is prevented by treatment with low-dosage estrogen with calcium', *Annals of Internal Medicine*, 1987, 106: 40–45.

Freedman, B.R. & Woodward, S. 'Behavioral treatment of menopausal hot flushes: evaluation by ambulatory monitoring', *American Journal of Obstetrics and Gynecology*, 1992, 167(2): 436–439.

Frontera, Walter R. et al. 'Strength conditioning in older men: skeletal muscle hypertrophy and improved function', *Journal of Applied Physiology*, 1988, vol 64: 1038–44.

Fu, S. 'Cross-cultural menopausal experience: a comparison of Australian and Tawainese women', unpublished Masters thesis, Queensland University of Technology, 2000

Gannon, L. 'Menopausal symptoms as consequences of dysrhythmia', *Journal of Behavioural Medicine*, 1993, Aug. 16(4): 387–402

Gilbert, R. *Bits and Pieces*, New Jersey: The Economic Press, 1999

Goldin, B.R., Aldercreutz, H., Gorbach, S.L. et al. 'The relationship between estrogen levels and diets of Caucasian American and Oriental immigrant women', *American Journal of Clinical Nutrition*, 1986, 44:945–953

Gordan, H. 'The correlation of menopausal symptoms with cytohormonal status', in

S. Cambell, *The Management of the Menopause and Postmenopausal Years*, Lancaster, MTP Press, 1976, 263–270

Greene, J.G., Cooke, D.J. 'Life stress and symptoms at the climacterium', *British Journal of Psychiatry*, 1980, 136:486–491

Griggs, R. *Personal Wellness*, Los Altos: Crisp Publications, 1990

Hammar, M., Berg, C. & Lindgren, R. 'Does physical exercise influence the frequency of postmenopausal hot flushes?', *Acta Obstetrica Et Gynecologia Scandinavia*, 1990, 69: 409–412.

Holte, A., Mikkelsen A. 'A factor-analyis study of climacteric symptoms', *Psychiatry and Social Science*, 1982, 2:35–39

Hulley, S., Grady, D., Bush, T., Furberg, C., Herrington, D., Riggs, B. & Vittinghoff, E. for the Heart and Estrogen/Progestin Replacement Study (HERS) Research Group. 'Randomized trial of estrogen plus progestin for secondary prevention of coronary heart disease in postmenopausal women', JAMA, 1998, 280:605–18

Hunter, M., Battersby, R., Whitehead, M. 'Relationships between psychological symptoms, somatic complaints and menopausal status', *Maturitas*,1986, 8: 217–88

Husband, A.J. 'Red clover isoflavone supplements: safety and pharmokinetics', *Journal of the British Menopause Society*, Supplement S1, 2001–04–20

Ingram, D., Sanders, K., Kolybaba, M. & Lopez, D. 'Case-control study of phyto-oestrogens and breast cancer', *Lancet*, 1997, 350:990–4

International Agency for Research on Cancer, 'Hormonal contraception and post-menopausal hormone therapy', Monographs on the Evaluation of Carcinogenic Risks to Humans, vol 72, Lyon: IARC, 1999

International Menopause Society, 'The International Menopause Society develops consensus clincial recommendations regarding hormone replacement therapy and heart disease: important Press Release', Royal Society of Medicine, London, 16 Oct., 2000

Kanis, J.A., Melton, L.J., Christiansen, C. et al. 'The diagnosis of osteoporosis', *Journal of Bone Mineral Rescue* 1994, 9:1137–41

Kaufert, P., & Gilbert, P. 'The context of menopause: psychotropic drug use and menopausal status', *Social Science Medicine*, 1984, 23: 747–755

Kaufert, P., Gilbert, P. & Tate, R. 'The Manitoba Project: a re-examination of the link between menopause and depression', *Maturitas*, 1992, 14(2): 143–156

Knight, D.C., Wall, P.L. & Eden, J.A. 'A review of phytoestrogens and their effects in relation to menopausal symptoms', *Australian Journal of Nutrition and Dietetics*, 1996, 53(1): 5–11

Koster, A. 'Change-of-life anticipations, attitudes and experiences among middle-aged Danish women', *Health Care Women International*, 1991, 12: 1–13

Law, M.R., Wald, N.J., & Meade, T.W. 'Strategies for prevention of osteoporosis and hip fracture', *British Medical Journal*, 1991, 303: 453–59

Lindsay, R. 'Sex steroids in the pathogenesis and prevention of osteoporosis', in B.I. Riggs (ed.), *Osteoporosis: Etiology, Diagnosis and Management*, New York, Raven Press, 1988: 333.

Lindsay, R. Hart, D.M., Forrest, C. & Baird, C. 'Prevention of spinal osteoporosis in oopherectomised women', *Lancet* 1980, 2:1151–3

Lock, M. 'Contested meaning of the menopause', *Lancet*, 1991, 337: 1270–3

Matthews, K.A. et al. 'Influences of natural menopause on psychological characteristics and symptoms of middle-aged healthy women', *Journal of Consulting and Clinical Psychology*, 1990, 58:345–351

McKinlay, S.M. & Jeffreys, M. 'The menopausal syndrome', *British Journal of Preventative Social Medicine*, 1974, 28: 108–115

McLennan, A.H. et al. 'Prevalence and cost of alternative medicine in Australia', *Lancet*, 1996, 347:569–73

Miller, A.B. & Bulbrook, R.D. 'The epidemiology, aetiology and prevention of breast cancer', *International Journal of Cancer*, 1986, 37: 173–177

Mizunuma, H., Okano, H., Soda, M. et al. 'Prevention of post-menopausal bone loss with minimal uterine blooding using low dose continuous estrogen/progestin therapy: a 2–year prospective study', *Maturitas*, 1997, 27: 69–76

Montero, I., Ruiz, I., & Hernandez, I. 'Social functioning as a significant factor in women's help-seeking behaviour during the climacteric period', *Social Psychiatry and Psychiatric Epidemiology*, 1993, 28, 178–183

Nachtigall, N.E., Nachtigall, R.H., Nachtigall, R.D., & Beckman, E.M. 'Estrogen replacement therapy: a 10-year prospective study in the relationship to osteoporosis', *Obstetrica and Gynaecology* 1979, 53: 277–81

National Health and Medical Research Council (NHMRC), *Menopause and Hormone Replacement Therapy: A Booklet for Women*, Commonwealth of Australia, 1999

NBCC 1999 'Breast self-examination and breast awareness: a summary of evidence for health professionals', Sydney: NBCC

Nelson, M.E. & Wernick, S. *Strong Women Stay Young*, Melbourne: Griffin Press 1997

Nelson, M.E. et al. 'Effects of high-intensity strength training on multiple risk factors for osteoporotic fractures: a randomized controlled trial', *Journal of the American Medical Association*, 1994, vol 272: 1909–14.

Notelovitz, M. et al. 'Estrogen therapy and variable-resistance weight training increase bone mineral in surgically menopausal women', *Journal of Bone and Mineral Research*, 1991, 6: 583–590.

Potter, S.M. et al. 'Effects of soy protein and isoflavones on plasma lipid profiles in postmenopausal women', *Second International Symposium on the Role of Soy in Preventing and Treating Chronic Disease*. Sept. 1006 (abstract)

Punyahotra, S. & Limpaphayom, K. 'An Asian perspective of the menopause', in *Progress in the Management of the Menopause* B. Wren (ed.), The Proceedings of the 8th International Congress on the Menopause, New York: The Parthenon Publishing Group, 1997

Recker, R.R., Saville, P.D. & Heaney, R.P. 'Effects of estrogens and calcium carbonate on bone loss in post-menopausal women', *Annals of Internal Medicine*, 1977, 87:649–55

Samselle, C. M., Messer, K.L., Herzog, A.R., Hines, S.H., Karl, C.R., Dioko, A.C., 'Effectiveness of classrom instruction in behavioural modification for urinary incontinence prevention', Women's Health and Menopause Conference proceedings, Washington DC, 19–23 May, 2001, 20

Sapsford, R., Bullock-Saxton, J., Markwell, S. *Women's Health: A Textbook for Physiotherapists*, London: WB Saunders Company Ltd, 1998

Shelton, R. 'St John's Wort ineffective for depression in first major trial' *JAMA*, 2001, 285:1978–1986

Standing, T.S. & Glazer, G. 'Attitudes of low income clinic patients toward menopause', *Health Care Women International*, 1992, 13: 271–280

Stanton, R. *Friendly Food*, Sydney, Murdoch Books, 1992

Stephens, F.O. 'Phytoestrogens and prostate cancer: possible preventive role', *The Medical Journal of Australia*, Aug. 1997, 167(3):138–140

Stewart F. 'The role of oestrogen as a lipid lowering agent', *Australasian Menopause Society Annual Congress Conference Program*, Oct. 1998

Stoppard, M. *Menopause*, Ringwood: Viking, 1994

Sturdee, D. (ed.) *HRT and Thromoembolism*, Royal Society of Medicine Press, London, 1997

Taylor, M. 'Dong Quai', Healthcare Reality Check FAQ Sheet, 2001 www.hcrc.org/faqs/dongquai.html

Thompson, B., Hart, S.A & Durno, D. 'Menopausal age and symptomatolgoy in a general practice', *Journal of Biosocial Science,* 1973, 5: 71–82

Utian, W.H. 'The true clinical features of post-menopause and oophorectomy and their response to oestrogen therapy', *South African Medical Journal*, 1972, 46: 732–737

Van Hall, E.V., Verdal, M. & Van der Velden, J. 'Perimenopausal complaints in women and men: a comparative study', *Journal of Women's Health*, 1994, 3: 45–49

Wilson, R.A., & Wilson, T.A. 'The fate of the nontreated postmenopausal woman: a plea for the maintenance of adequate estrogen from puberty to the grave', *Journal of the American Geriatric Society*, 1963, 11: 347

Wilson, R.A., Brevetti, R.E. & Wilson, T.A. 'Specific procedures for the elimination of the menopause', *Western Journal of Surgical Obstetrics and Gynecology*, 1963, 7: 110

Wimalawansa, S.J. 'A four-year randomised controlled trial of hormone replacement and bisphosphonate, alone or in combination, in women with post-menopausal osteoporosis', *American Journal of Medicine* 1998, 104 219–216

World Health Organization, *Sixth Report on the World Health Situation*, Part 1, Global Analysis, Geneva, 1980

World Health Organization, *Research on the Menopause in the 1990s: Report of a WHO Scientific Group*, Geneva, 1996

Wren, B.G. 'Megatrials of hormonal replacement therapy', *Changes*, 1998, 98:3

Zhang, J., Feldblum, P. J. & Fortney, J.A. 'Moderate physical activity and bone density among perimenopausal women', *American Journal of Public Health*, 82 (5) May 1992: 736–8.

Index

abdominal curling machine 94
abdominals 93–4
  bracing 93
  curlups 93–4
aerobic exercise 84–6, 110, 111
ageing 16–17
  related symptoms 10, 18–19
alcohol 46, 51, 64
alternative medicine 149
American Cancer Society 137
anxiety 132, 133

baby boomers 6–7
back problems 23, 95, 110, 118
balance 73, 77, 79, 87
bicep curl 98
black cohosh 160, 164
bladder control 22, 103–5
bleeding
  breakthrough 131
  irregular 23
blood pressure, high 60, 80, 81
blood sugar level 46
body shape 58, 79–80
bone loss 28, 30, 47, 75, 77

bone mineral density 29–30, 31, 74, 87, 139
  and HRT 138–40
bones 73–4, 139
  and exercise 73–6
  life cycle 74
bread 63
  soy/linseed 53, 56, 69
breakfast 57, 62
breakthrough bleeding 131
breast cancer 32–3, 54, 55, 135, 155
  and HRT 135–6, 138, 146
  prevention 33–4, 53
  study 133–4
breast self-examination 33, 34
breast tenderness 131
BreastScreen Australia 33, 34

caffeine 31, 40, 46, 51
calcium 47–9, 69, 73–4, 139
  absorption 50–2
  amount in food 49–50
  and exercise 75–6
  RDI 47
  supplements 52–3

cancer 53, 55, 124, 135–8, 155
  see also breast cancer
carbohydrates 46
cardiovascular disease (CVD) 25–8,
    80–1, 135, 155
  checklist 26
  and HRT 140–1
  and phytoestrogens 55
  prevention 28
  study 133–4
cardiovascular exercise 84–6, 110, 111
cervical cancer 137
cholesterol 25–6, 42, 43, 60, 80, 81
  HDL 42, 43, 55
  LDL 26, 42, 43, 55
clinical trials 10
coffee 40, 46
colorectal cancer 53, 137–8
complementary medicine 149–51, 161
  choosing a practitioner 152
  problems 150–2
  websites 153
complex carbohydrates 46
concentration, lack of 19, 23, 132
confidence 73, 82–3
consultations, with GP 7, 126–7,
    131–2, 152
cookbooks 61
coronary heart disease 25, 43, 60
coumarins 159, 160
coumestans 53, 54, 156
cross-sectional studies 133, 141

dairy products 44, 46
  calcium content 49, 50
deep vein thrombosis (DVT) 25, 131–2,
    140
dehydration 40, 41
dementia 142
depression 19, 23, 36, 83, 132–3, 161–2
diabetes, adult-onset 60, 80, 81–2
diet 9, 27, 154, 168
  fat intake 41–5
  freshness 44, 45
  guidelines 39
  high-fat foods 44
  low-fat foods 44, 49

variety 45, 62
water 39–41, 107
  see also fats
dietary supplements 52
dieting 59–60, 70
dinner 57, 64
diuretics 40
dizziness 19, 23, 132
doctors 125–7, 150, 151, 152
  and communication 7, 126–7
dong quai 159–60
dumbbells 95

eating plan 38, 39, 65, 68
  see also diet
education 13
  see also research, personal
endometrial cancer 53, 55, 124
  and HRT 136–7, 138
endorphins 83
energy 46, 59, 78
  lack of 19, 23, 132
epidemiological data 157
evening primrose oil 161
exercise 16, 21, 27, 72–3, 154, 164, 169
  and balance 77, 79
  benefits 73–83, 117, 118
  and calcium 75–6
  cardiovascular (aerobic) 84–6, 110,
    111
  checkpoints 115–16
  and emotional well-being 82–3
  getting started 108–16
  and metabolism 59
  muscle strength 77–9
  and osteoporosis 31
  plans 113–15
  reps/sets 88
  strong bones 73–6
  and water 40
  weight control 79–80
exercises
  with dumbbells 96–9
  in fitness centre 100
  lower back 95
  no equipment 87–95

fall prevention 31
fats 41–3, 140
  bad 42
  in diet, reducing 44
  good 42, 43
  monounsaturated 41, 42
  omega 3 fatty acids 42, 43
  polyunsaturated 42
  saturated 41, 42
feminism 6
fibre 46, 52
fish 43, 50, 63
fitness centres 99–100, 111
fitness trainers 111, 112
flavones 156
flexibility 100–2
fluid retention 19, 23, 58, 132
fractures 28–30, 47, 79, 138, 139–40
  risk factors 28–9
frequency see urinary problems
fruit 45–6, 50, 64

general practitioners (GPs) 7, 125–7,
  150, 151, 152
genetics 5, 9, 30, 81
ginseng 160

Harvard Women's Health Watch 15
headaches 19, 23
health
  chronic conditions 14–15
  information 14–15, 126, 151, 168
  self-rated 13–14, 16
heart disease see cardiovascular disease
Heart and Estrogen–Progestin
  Replacement Study (HERS) 134,
  140–1, 216
herbs 151, 159
high-fat foods 44
hope 166
hormone replacement therapy (HRT) 3,
  24, 58, 123–6, 150
  and bone loss 31
  and the brain 142
  and breast cancer 135–6, 138
  and calcium 48

and cervical cancer 137
and colorectal cancer 137–8
and CVD 140–1
and endometrial cancer 136–7, 138
and hot flushes 20, 130
long-term 129–30, 133–4, 145
and osteoporosis 138–40
and ovarian cancer 137
prescription-only 125–6
psychological health 132–3
research studies 133–4
short-term 129, 130–2, 144
use 127–8
hot flushes 19–21, 36, 54–5, 102
  and HRT 20, 130
  and phytoestrogens 20, 22, 54–5
HRT see hormone replacement therapy
  (HRT)
hysterectomy 125, 131

incontinence 103–5, 107, 118
insomnia 19, 23, 130
intercourse, uncomfortable 21
International Menopause Society 141
isoflavones 53, 54, 55–6, 156
  intakes compared by country 156

Jan's story 65–7
Juliet's story 14

lactose 51
legumes 53, 54
life expectancy 6
lifestyle 9, 27
  risk factors 27
lifestyle diseases 53, 80–2
lignans 53, 54, 156
linseed 53, 54, 56
longitudinal studies 133, 136, 141
low-fat foods 44, 49
lower back exercises 95
lunch 57, 63–4
lunges 89–90, 97

mammograms 33, 34
meat 44, 52
meditation 15, 102

menopause 3, 4–5, 36
  and symptoms 12–13, 18–19
  average age 6
  cross-cultural 8–10, 20, 21
  deficiency disease 6, 8, 17
  early 130, 131
  expectations 8, 168
  negative perceptions 5–6
  outside influences 10–11
  positive attitude 11, 16–17, 82
Menopause Made Simple Program 2, 4,
  11, 27, 167–70
menstruation 12, 23
  irregular 19, 23
metabolism 58–9, 60, 62, 78, 80
Million Women Study 134, 136, 216
mobility 51, 77
monounsaturated fats 41, 42
muscle mass 59, 60, 77–8
muscle strength 73, 77–9, 87

Natural Alternatives to HRT Cookbook 57
natural progesterone 157–8, 164
nervous tension 19, 20, 23, 132, 133
night sweats 19–21, 36
  and HRT 130
nipple change 33
Novogen 164
nutritional labels 44–5

oestrogen 58, 80, 104, 124, 125
  and bone loss 28
oestrogen-only therapy 125, 136, 146
oils 44, 62, 64
omega 3 fatty acids 42, 43
osteoblasts 74
osteoclasts 74
osteopenia 74
osteoporosis 28–30, 55, 74–5
  checklist 29
  and HRT 138–40
  prevention 30–2
  risk factors 75
  study 133–4
ovarian cancer 137

paced respiration 21
palpitations 19, 23, 132
peak bone mass 31
pelvic floor exercises 23, 94, 105–7
perimenopause 23
personal fitness trainers 111, 112
phytochemicals 53–7
phytoestrogens 9, 20, 53–7, 154–7
  and hot flushes 20, 22, 54–5
  sources 156
  supplements 154–5, 156, 157
polyunsaturated fats 42
Postmenopausal Estrogen/Progestin
  Intervention (PEPI) Trial 134,
  140, 215–16
premenstrual tension (PMT) 4
progesterone 125
  natural 157–8, 164
progestogen 124, 157
Promensil 156
prostate cancer 53, 155
protein 52
pushups, modified 90–1, 97

red clover 53, 156
Rejuvex 160
relaxation 15, 82, 102
Remifemin 160
research, personal 5, 10, 13, 14–15, 126
research findings 125
research methods
  clinical trials 10
  cross-sectional studies 133, 141
  epidemiological studies 157
  longitudinal studies 133, 136, 141
research studies, HRT 133–4
respiration, paced 21

St John's wort 161–2
salad dressing 63
salt 46, 51
Sandra's story 111–13
sandwiches 63
saturated fats 41, 42
self-esteem 13, 73, 82–3
self-rated health 13–14, 16

sexual activity 21
sexual interest, decreased 22, 158
shopping list 61
shoulder press 97–8
simple carbohydrates 46
sleep problems 19, 23, 130
smoking 15–16, 20, 27, 51
snacks 57, 64–5
soy 53, 54, 55, 56, 69, 154
squats 88–9, 96
starches 46
strength 77–8
strength training 78–9, 87–8, 110, 111,
    119
stress 15, 18–19, 80, 82, 102, 154
  management strategies 15, 82
stretches
  chest 101
  gluteals 101
  hamstring 100
  quadricep 101
  shoulder 101
stretching 86, 100–2
stroke 25
sugars 46
supplements 52

testosterone 125
thrombosis see deep vein thrombosis
    (DVT)
tofu 54, 56, 154
tricep dips, seated 91–2
tricep extension, overhead 99
triglycerides 26

urgency see urinary problems
urinary problems 21, 22–3, 103–5
urinary system 103–4

vaginal dryness 54–5, 104
  and HRT 21, 130
vaginal wall, changes to 20, 21–2
vegetables 45–6, 50
venous thromboembolism see deep vein
    thrombosis (DVT)
vitamin D 50–1, 139

walking 85, 86, 111
water, in the body 39–41, 107
water-based activities 76, 110
weight control 27, 58–62
  exercise 79–80
  and water 40–1
weight gain 58, 60, 69–70, 80
  and HRT 132, 146
weight training see strength training
weight-bearing activities 76, 85
wholegrains 45–6
wild yam cream 159, 164
women
  attitudes to 9, 17
  life expectancy 6
Women's Health Initiative 134, 136,
    215
Women's International Study of Long
    Duration Oestrogen after
    Menopause (WISDOM) 134, 216
Women's Waterworks: Curing Incontinence
    107
World Health Organization (WHO) 6,
    10, 18–19, 48, 135, 136

yoga 15, 102